INFERTILITY MADNESS

One Couple's Journey Through Infertility Hell

ALEX HARLE

AND

JASON GIBBS

The moral rights of the authors, to be identified as such, has been asserted in accordance with the Copyright, Designs and Patents Act 1988.

This book details the authors' personal experiences with and opinions about infertility. It is not making any recommendations about any medical treatments. The authors are not medically trained. In fact, they are the very opposite (and particularly Alex who is a numpty when it comes to the sciences) so please, if anything, utterly ignore everything they say and follow your own path, get your own medical advice, decide for yourself what is best for you. The point of this book is simply to show that someone else has been on this journey and survived to tell the tale. Its aim is really to show the toll infertility takes, particularly in relation to mental health and if it can, offer a few rays of light.

ISBN: 9798710132029

For the GBs and the IFs

**"Insanity is doing the same thing over and over
again and expecting different results."**

Albert Einstein, or maybe Rita Mae Brown,

or maybe Alcoholics Anonymous

THE FEMALE PERSPECTIVE

1

In the Beginning

"The journey of a thousand miles begins with one step."

Lao Tzu

If someone had told me 10 years ago I would have considered suicide on an almost daily basis for well over a year, desperately wanted to self-harm even though I didn't have the stomach for it, was so utterly consumed by anger and despair, utterly unable to think about anything else for literally what seemed like every waking moment, that I would demolish, by brute force and rage, three vacuum cleaners, a dishwasher, a tumble dryer, one laptop and part of an oak floor I would not have believed it. Not for a minute.

Not me; I had it all: married at 27 to an amazing, loving husband, well-paid and challenging job, big house in the country, loving parents. I even had Labradors. I thought that "kind of stuff" happened to other people. Only people who weren't strong enough to deal with life needed counselling. Not me; and certainly not then on to a faith healer. I went to one of those schools – the ones where they ingrain you with the belief that you can do anything; you just have to put your mind to it. And I did. For a long time.

Standing in the shower one morning, the warmish water running down, I was thinking about trying to explain how it felt to be infertile to the latest doctor we were seeing. Should I go with it being a bit like one of those fairground rides from the old days with the toy on elastic string that you have to try and catch as the carousel goes round? It swings and jerks erratically; tantalisingly close and yet always out of reach. It's always some other lucky kid going home with the highly prized soft toy.

Or that it's like some kind of sick hide and seek game in a maze, against the clock? If you navigate your way through there is a beautiful bouncing baby waiting for you. Along the way you will be given snippets of advice, some of which is contradictory, some of which is plain bonkers, but still, you just never know, so, in your desperate search, you try and follow all of it anyway, just in case. Unless you can decipher the truth and find the right path through the maze, the baby will be lost forever. And, always, in the background, the clock is ticking down. Tick, tock, tick, tock. On and on it goes.

Had someone told me that there were dangers in leaving it too late; in living a certain lifestyle, in pushing myself to the limit in everything I did, I very much doubt I would have changed anything. I'm not sure I was capable of changing. But, and it is a big but, maybe it would have hit home. That maybe, just maybe, I couldn't actually have it all, at least not all at the same time. That how you live your life does have consequences.

This book is about how not to do things; it is a note of lessons learned and a bloody good kick up the arse (which I am still trying to give myself). I spent 6, no, make that nearly 7, years of my life desperately, desperately trying to get pregnant and when I repeatedly failed, wallowing in bitterness, pain and anger.

Some of this story comes from a diary I kept during IVF cycles so is pretty detailed. The rest is often a summary or just random thoughts along the way.

If anyone is reading this, don't be surprised if you don't like me. I didn't either for much of the time. But if even one line or thought helps you then I will consider it a job well done. I also just want to apologise for the swearing. I have removed a lot of it from previous drafts but quite a bit still remains, because, quite frankly, it seemed to me the situation warranted it. So if swearing puts you off, please don't read any further.

2

The Start

"Start by doing the necessary, then what's possible; and suddenly you are doing the impossible."

Saint Francis of Assisi

I always wanted children. Not in the way that some girls want a big white wedding and go slowly insane planning for the big day before an even vaguely Mr. Right appears on the scene but rather I had just assumed (positively) that I would have children. One day. It is, after all, or so it seemed to me, the natural order of things. So it would happen; when I was ready.

By 30, I was ready. Well, more accurately, at 30, a fucking bomb went off. Not only was I ready but my entire body and mind were screaming for a child. My friends were all pregnant or already popped (or at least so it seemed). Babies and bumps everywhere. How hard could it be? Right? I was thinking a Summer baby would be lovely so that meant Autumn was the best time to try. I was thinking maternity leave, buying lovely things for the baby, I literally had visions of myself skipping along through a field of straw with the pram, sun shining, a gentle breeze blowing as the baby sleeps.

So, it was time, it was time to get on with it. Everything I had learnt in sex education classes (all two of them) was that you can get pregnant at the drop of a hat; take the pill 30 minutes late and be in the same room as someone of the opposite sex and there would be a sproglet on the way before you know it.

And yet, for me, there had always been a nagging feeling, tucked away in the back of my mind that things wouldn't be quite that straightforward.

I was born with a congenital hip disorder, but several operations later, as well as traction for six months, frog-plaster and callipers I was not just able to walk in a straight line but also run everywhere. My parents often told me the story of how, even with plaster from my armpits to my ankles (with a convenient hole for a nappy to be "tucked in") I would drag myself everywhere, up and down the stairs, up and down sandy beaches. So I guess the stubbornness, and utter refusal to take any account of things which might otherwise have held me back, was there from the beginning. So, it was great when I could finally run unimpeded; but then other things popped up. By 14 I was wetting myself every time I did run. Sometimes a warm trickle running down my legs, other times just damp knickers. There is something about damp knickers. Like it is a dark, dirty secret. Can you get home and change before anyone spots it or smells it? Running, good. Stress incontinence, not so good. Anyway. Despite three operations for incontinence between 14 and 21, the leaks didn't stop.

So, not surprisingly, that whole area seemed like a mess to me. Add to that that I had never been able to use applicator tampons (they just didn't seem to work) and I guess I was looking for problems from the start.

Plus sex hurt. A lot.

But sex was required for babies (according to those ever informative sex education lessons) so sex it was. Slow, fast, blitz. Every day, every other day, with cough medicine, without cough medicine, when the little ovulation machine said yes, even if the ovulation machine said no; just in case.

Actually at one point we followed the "sperm meets egg plan":

1. Day 8 to Ovulation: every other night
2. Test for ovulation from Day 10 onwards
3. Ovulation onwards: every night for three nights, then not on the fourth night, then on the fifth night
4. If no apparent ovulation: every other night until day 35
   Note: release sperm at least once between ovulation and the next cycle.

That went on for 3 months. Nothing.

So then it was the cough medicine programme:

1. Take cough medicine every day, a few hours before sex.
2. Have sex every day from day 10 until ovulation.

That went on for another three months. Nothing.

I was starting to panic. The "advice" from friends, the internet, everyone so it seemed – carry on for at least nine months, better still a year; don't worry about it; and, of course, my favourite, the words that would ring in my ears for the next six years: "just relax"; it'll happen, all in good time. Jason, my husband, was firmly in that category – all we needed was to have lots of sex and you, highly strung wife, need to relax and all will be well. But I don't work like that (just leaving things alone, letting them be) and every period, every month, didn't feel like I was getting any closer to being pregnant; rather the opposite, it felt like it was getting further away, becoming an impossibility.

It was time to do something.

3

The Scourge of Endometriosis

"I can't change the direction of the wind, but I can adjust my sails to always reach my destination."

Jimmy Dean

Dr Fake Tan (as he shall henceforth be known) alternated between tapping various parts of my abdomen and poking around internally, "Yes, that hurts; yes, that hurts too". On it went. I lay there, knickers off, legs apart – far beyond the point of having any dignity (having already told him that it hurt when I had sex; yes, sometimes I bleed from sex and yes, you know, it does put me off it a bit; yes, I would really rather have sex at night, just before I go to sleep because at least then there is some chance I can sleep through the worst of the pain).

Now Dr Fake Tan was an interesting one, a Monet shall we say. He looked the real deal from the outside – tanned, good-looking, highly recommended (by my GP at least). But as it turned out not actually the best doctor when it came to imparting information.

Lesson no.1: listen very, very carefully to every single word when you are in front of a doctor. Better still, take detailed notes or take someone with you to listen. Even better than that, turn your phone on to record. This is important for two reasons. First, the brains of most people tend to go to mush in front of doctors talking about their own medical issues (for some utterly ridiculous and infuriating reason). Number two, some doctors – like everyone else, may have a tendency to gloss over the truth; to not answer the question you asked; to answer questions they would rather answer; to ignore you entirely and just give you their "sales" patter/tell you the things they do know.

That brings us to **Lesson no. 2**: most (okay, the vast majority by my reckoning) of the doctors in the field of infertility don't know very much. This is also for two reasons. Number one: the science surrounding fertility is still very basic (although there have been some amazing advances, such as IVF itself). Number two: the science can be very basic, because of that very advance of IVF. In my experience, infertility "specialists" will rarely ask you a question about your health, your lifestyle, your partner's health etc. They don't need to. All they need are the results to some very basic tests/questions – How old are you? What is your AMH (Anti-Mullerian Hormone)? When was your last period? Have you completed our vast array of consent forms? And last, but most importantly, can you afford it? The answer is then IVF, ICSI or some other equivalent.

Back to Dr Fake Tan. He looked like the finished article – a caring man who clearly knew his stuff and would, if I believed him, have a baby inside me in two shakes of a lamb's tail (not personally, obviously).

To be fair, Dr Fake Tan diagnosed endometriosis. Get this, blood cells grow inside of you, in places other than the uterus and then, when you bleed during your period, the additional rogue blood cells also bleed. They could be in your nose, your arm, your stomach. Anywhere. The blood may be able to escape or it may not.

I was lucky. Although the pain during my period was relatively severe, the endometriosis was not. All it required, apparently, was a laparoscopy by the charming Dr Fake Tan to check he was right, a further operation to remove it (and cauterise parts of my cervix) and I would be good to go. That actually meant a stay in hospital, a general anaesthetic, a day off work. It's probably not the right thing to say but given things were so crazy (I was working 14-hour days, had a 4-hour commute, lived in an unfinished barn conversion and we had a smallholding with about 70 animals to look after), a general anaesthetic, i.e. some guaranteed "sleep" and a day off the treadmill sounded amazing to me. Just to be clear, when I say "unfinished barn conversion", it wasn't that the place needed a lick of paint. The previous inhabitants, the cows, had moved out of 7 weeks before we moved in. We therefore lived in a make-shift "house" within the barn, with a chipboard floor balanced on bricks to lift us away from the cow urine-soaked floor. Despite having moved in in January, for some reason we thought roof insulation was optional, there were holes in the walls, holes in the roof, rats running around. So now I think about it, probably not the best environment to be trying to bring a child into but hey, I was going for a Summer baby so all would be well by then.

The operation went well. But try and ask Dr Fake Tan a question – what does endometriosis mean for my chances of getting pregnant? Is there anything else I can do to stop it coming back? How did I get it in the first place? When can I start trying again? The man quite literally ran away; out of the room, without giving a single coherent answer.

Five months later. The pain was still there, so he had another go – this time to laser the endometriosis.   Better luck this time around; we were hoping... So another general anaesthetic, another hospital stay, some more time off work although, as I now knew, missing more work just meant there would be more late nights to come as I sought to catch up. But my overwhelming feeling was that the doctors could do whatever they liked. A bag hanging out of me draining blood away, another few scars, no problem, as long as I was on the way to getting pregnant.

4

Needling and Chinese

"Patience is a bitter plant, but its fruit is sweet."

Chinese Proverb

By the time I had finished trying to get the endometriosis sorted almost a year had passed since we had first started trying. Nothing. It was time to try another tack. Needles, or more accurately, acupuncture.

Based on a recommendation from a friend I went to see an acupuncturist in London. In very marked contrast to Dr Fake Tan, she took a lot of details about my periods, the pain, the clots, the varying cycle length. Then she popped a number of needles in and left me to stew. The hardest thing was just lying there. The only other time I did "nothing" was when I slept so this just felt wrong and also slightly nerve-wracking:

"What if she doesn't come back?"

"What if she forgets about me?"

"What is she doing?"

But she did always come back and slowly my periods began to change, the clots became smaller, the cycle shortened. I had been pretty sceptical about acupuncture but the physical results and changes were undeniable.

For some time prior to all this infertility malarkey, I had been seeing a Chinese doctor (Dr Blunt as she will henceforth be called) on the edge of China Town in London to treat urticaria, which I had been suffering from for years. To be fair, over a long period of time it was getting better despite the fact that during the vast majority of that time I had no faith that the dodgy black little pills in plastic bags I was handed each week were anything other than placebos. The same went for the crazy, stinky herb mixture (boil it down, stink your house out, wonder what the hell you are doing variety) which she "prescribed" from time to time.

However, at one appointment when I mentioned I was trying to get pregnant she told me, in that beautifully blunt way she had, "it will take a long time, start charting your temperature". Oh and, "send your husband for a sperm test". Oh, and last but not least, "even if you do get pregnant now, you will miscarry". My body, according to her, was not in a fit state to receive a baby. I felt shocked and hurt, as if her words had physically punched me, but as I was to find out, she was absolutely right.

Not that I had even heard of them at that stage but temperature charts it therefore was. In time, I came to hate them; really, really hate them. Had

I lain still enough?   How can I lie still and still reach out for the thermometer which I have stupidly managed to knock onto the floor?

The charts measure temperature, cervical mucus (dry, wet, stretchy, crumbly and creamy), blood colour (dark red, average (whatever the hell that means) bright red and brown), blood clots (small or large), volume of blood loss (starting with "flood" down to "low"), level of pain (high, medium or low).

On and on they went.

Jason did go for a sperm test. It showed high abnormal forms and a repeat test was recommended. Dr Blunt also informed me Jason should have a blood test. He refused. Point blank. Personally, blood tests had never been a problem for me. As far as I was concerned, they could take the lot as long as it provided an answer. What I didn't appreciate at the time was that he basically had a phobia about them. So instead of a blood test she prescribed some more vile smelling herbs to boil and imbibe, for him this time. Presumably a general catch all for what may or may not have been revealed in the blood test.

Despite all the needling, the little black placebos, the herbs, the "pep" talks from Dr Blunt, the two operations, the problem remained. Not even a hint of pregnancy.

Around the same time Jason was travelling back and forth to the US for work and his Dad's cancer had returned. We knew how much it would mean to his Dad to have grandchildren but as with all the fertility stuff, despite desperately pushing for treatments as quickly as possible we were ultimately helpless, watching on as the cancer progressed and the clock wound down. Then one Friday the call came. Jason had just landed in the US as his Dad had tragically passed away. I rushed from work to be with my mother-in-law and Jason got straight back on a plane knowing it was all too late.

Still, two years in and now too late for his Dad to ever see grandchildren, we pushed on and it was back to our local fertility centre.

This time, for our first encounter with Dr Relax (so called because apart from so kindly "allowing" us to do IVF, his steadfast advice remained that all I needed to do was change my entire lifestyle and just "relax"). To double check the endometriosis was still not causing any problems, he performed the same procedure as Dr Fake Tan, just with messier stitching (his irritated comment, not mine). It turns out even amongst fertility doctors there is professional jealousy. Weirdly, I thought the fact that Dr Fake Tan hadn't actually done the job properly, had an appalling bedside manner and failed to answer a single one of my questions was more important, but apparently not. Another laparoscopy, hysteroscopy and dye. Luckily, this one showed no endometriosis, which was good on the one hand but also not good in that it meant something else was going on.

4

Dr Perfect

"The greatest wisdom is seeing through appearances."

Atisa

Having despaired of Dr Fake Tan and Dr Relax, I decided London was the answer.

A number of friends (one of whom was pregnant with twins) extolled the virtues of a doctor on Harley Street. Let's call him Dr Perfect.

Money no barrier (at this stage all the endometriosis treatment had been covered on our private health insurance), I telephoned the hospital to which he was linked and got an appointment. Even better, Dr Perfect had "rooms" on Harley Street. Wow, he must be good. Or was it that he just charged so much he could afford to rent rooms on Harley Street.

Off we went.

I arrived for the appointment late, sweating profusely, having literally run nearly all the way up Harley Street, which as it turned out was bloody long. Panic about the damp knickers thing was starting to kick in. Jason, the epitome of calm, was, of course, already there – waiting outside, relaxed, coffee in hand. So, we were late but that was okay because the doctor was even later (is that a power game thing or what?). But that was actually good because it gave the sweat, and the knickers, a chance to dry out.

Finally, we were ushered in. Dr Perfect was the consummate professional. He explained the science behind various things, listened to my explanation of endometriosis (as I surreptitiously tried to wipe the final bits of sweat away), and offered tests. He had an extremely knowing air, jotting down the odd word with his expensive fountain pen and looking at us confidently from behind his vast mahogany desk. From memory I even managed not to cry. Which was pretty much a first.

Tests it was and Jason finally agreed to a blood test and a sperm test, me to a range of blood tests. Thankfully because of the endometriosis, it appeared that most bills, certainly the initial investigatory ones would be also covered by our health insurer.

A few days later, we were back in the plush waiting rooms. It was an exact re-run – me sweating like a pig, Jason calm and collected. Dr Perfect ran through the results. He was assurance and confidence personified. I could see why others trusted him – as did I at that stage. He carefully explained that whilst there did not appear to be any reason why I was not getting pregnant naturally the best way to find out would be a round of IVF. I didn't hear much more after that – finally, maybe this would be it. I'd never been one to worry about hospital procedures – so the process held no fear and it meant that SOMETHING WAS GOING TO BE DONE.

According to Dr Perfect, IVF offered a win-win. It would give us a decent shot at pregnancy (just by doing it) but it would also be diagnostic. The way the process worked, so we were told, would enable them to examine what was going on at each stage and therefore determine the part that was the problem. I either get pregnant from the process or I get an answer which can then be fixed. Awesome.

Then it was on to Jason's test results. His semen analysis showed that he was "perfect"; no problem on his side.

"Perfect." Jason kept repeating it, out loud, as he literally skipped down the street. I could fuck off with my nagging over alcohol (I had screamed so loudly at him during one row that my throat hurt for two days); Jason had it on the very best authority (from someone with Dr before their name and rooms on Harley Street no less) that his sperm was PERFECT. That meant one thing and one thing only. All of this, the months of not getting pregnant, the fuss and the hassle, all of it, must be my fault.

It didn't really strike me then that the reason for the skipping and enormous grin plastered all over his face was that he had actually been worried it was him; that blanks were being fired.

I had always assumed all that masculine pride stuff just wasn't his thing. But, thinking about it now, it had never actually been tested.

The impression I had had up until that point was that Jason's overwhelming diagnosis of "our" situation was that I fuss and if I could just relax and have more sex then all of this ridiculous doctor, procedure, test nonsense would disappear (along with the exorbitant cost) and a bouncing baby would duly arrive. But maybe underneath it all, there had been a concern that actually it might be due to something on his side.

So, IVF it was (the antagonist protocol apparently). A few days later, the drugs arrived in a massive box, at work.

†

With a little help from my friends

Taking the big box of IVF drugs home on the train I bumped into Meredith, newly a mother. Meredith being Meredith, we talked about her. She actually knew I was thinking of IVF and I think I did mention the huge box contained the requisite drugs. At least I think I got to the end of that sentence. It would be hard to say as the next 30 minutes (until her stop) was consumed by her childcare concerns, issues with Doug not pulling his weight, not having a clue when it comes to parenting, the need to have the right car in which to transport her precious one, the right person to provide the right childcare, how to go about getting him into the right school (said child was only 9 months old at this point).

A week later it was Christine. We had both started trying at roughly the same time. Eight months later we were bemoaning the lack of progress. We shared our anger, upset, frustration. We talked about how difficult it was that everyone else seemed to be pregnant.

One month later, she was pregnant.

The next nine months were fucking hell – for both of us. Did I not know how hard it was to be pregnant? NO, I FUCKING DIDN'T. But she carried on, every month I failed to get pregnant, telling me what new item for the nursery she had just bought, how difficult it was to get a car seat that fits, how her skin itched, how tight her clothes were (which really didn't need to be said, as she followed the fashion for showing off her bump, so I could tell on a daily basis that they didn't fit, in fact I could tell she was the proud owner of an outy belly button). "BUY PROPER MATERNITY CLOTHES. ONES THAT FIT and don't make you look like you are wearing an oversized condom." I wanted to shout, every day, but somehow managed not to.

On one level I was genuinely, really happy for her. But on another level, I just wanted to scream, "please, just FUCK OFF, has baby brain wiped your memory of all our conversations and removed the last semblance of empathy? Go and speak to someone who isn't trying to get pregnant and who might actually give a shit."

Rant over, back to the IVF.

†

The actual process took place at the hospital linked to the clinic. We were, of course, late, despite thinking we had left a load a time in which to get lost and navigate the London traffic. So once more, we arrived late, arguing and then joy of joy, had to work out how to get to the fertility unit? It turned out the answer to that question was through the maternity ward, of course. SERIOUSLY. WHAT THE FUCK.

The place itself was like something out of a 70s horror movie, a cold, decrepit building, held together with sticky tape, chipped paint which flaked off as you walked past, stained curtains to each cubicle. Even the floor was sticky (I tried not to inspect with what). Jason went off to do his bit. Apparently, this part of the set up was trying to be state of the art – so they provided a video player no less, in place of the usual array of top shelf material. Yes, ok, their weird idea of state of the art was more like being stuck in the 70s but it utterly failed anyway because there were no actual videos.

The call came: eleven eggs collected, 5 diploid, 2 transploid; two average quality, one poor and the rest it would seem not even worth talking about. So, it turns out it is possible to be judged even before birth. But good enough for a day 3 transfer. Woohoo.

The day came and the first thing they did was hand us photos of the embryos in a little cardboard folder. You know you have entered some warped world when you get photos of the embryos still in their petri dish. I get the point – this could be the very first photo of your child/children. But it could also be (and is far more likely to be) another reminder of your abject failure.   Are you still supposed to keep it if the IVF fails, as a memento of the great times you had getting close to motherhood?

Transfer done, off we went home. To wait. Has it worked? Do I feel pregnant? Would you feel pregnant this early? Do I feel any different? Should I have just eaten that? It was endless. Every waking minute. Every time I went to the loo – was that blood? Was that pain, is that embryos embedding or period pain?

Ten days later, the answer came. I was in bed. Brown at first and then the red rush. Somewhere in there were the embryos. Then the pain. Emotional and physical. Searing. I curled up in bed, blood soaking through to the mattress.

The next day was Bank Holiday Monday but I still tried to call the helpline to ask what I was supposed to do. I kept punching at the phone keypad but I couldn't get the number to go through. In my torment and anguish I had actually been dialling the wrong digits but was incapable of realising what I was doing. I'm not sure why I bothered. By the time I spoke to someone they just said do nothing. I could almost hear the, "you've just become part of our failure rate, thanks for nothing".

Back we went to the clinic, for the post mortem (I guess literally). And do you know what, weirdly Dr Perfect was no longer talking about the win-win of IVF. He was no longer extolling the virtues of it being diagnostic.

He was no longer going to give us a longed for answer. In fact, there was no diagnosis; no diagnosis at all. The word didn't even appear in his monologue.

His finding? We had been unlucky. We just needed to roll the dice again. It was as if the clouds had suddenly parted. This wasn't science. This wasn't a targeted medical treatment. This certainly wasn't trying to find out what was wrong and fix it, to avoid IVF. This was a salesman, doing his job. He had to weigh up whether the odds of it working with a particular couple (and therefore keeping the clinic's stats high) were worth it. Clearly, we were a good enough bet that he was willing to let us pay him about £5,000 again. His job was to make sure that £5,000 was spent at his clinic and not elsewhere. He even joked that some other clinics have a better success rate on their waiting list than with their treatment. He did also mention that for three months after an IVF cycle you are supposed to be more fertile so we should take advantage of that – like it was some throw away freebie, "Spend a fortune on one IVF cycle, fail and you get three months super fertility for free". As if.

We said we'd think about it. Jason was angry. Mr Perfect was no longer so perfect. He couldn't or wouldn't provide any answers. He couldn't or wouldn't provide any stats.

All I knew was that I felt tired, worried, angry, frustrated, guilty, irrational but seemingly without the power to change any of that. I also felt angry but more than anything I felt fear, gut-wrenching fear – that I just couldn't get pregnant. Soon after we got married we had talked about children, and both of us had muttered that we'd love to have four. Four. What a joke. I was incapable of even one.

5

The Data-Based IVF

"He uses statistics as a drunken man uses lamp posts – for support rather than for illumination."

Andrew Lang

I think you can tell a lot about a place from its waiting rooms and our second IVF clinic (let's call it the Lainsborough) had about six and then various chairs in corridors. I spent an inordinate amount of time in those corridors. Waiting. And then some.

We initially liked the doctor at the Lainsborough. She seemed very sensible and, ridiculous as this may sound as a description of a doctor, scientific. As we had decided to give up on Dr Perfect, this was a godsend. As far as she was concerned (let's call her Dr Stats) trying to get pregnant is like continually throwing a dice but, with the Lainsborough as she assured us, each throw could be utterly refined, tweaked and scrutinised. It was all going to be about the data. To the extent possible, this was where nature met science. We could address the frustrations with Dr Perfect, and Jason seemed excited that there would, at last, be numbers.

So we had three choices:

i)   IUI – 12% success rate. Spin eggs and sperm together and shove in the womb. Cross fingers.

ii)   IVF – ovulate, produce eggs, fertilise outside of the womb, shove embryos back in. 1 in 3 chance.

iii)   Continue to try naturally.

Overall stats per cycle for IVF:

- Over 40: 20% chance

- 30-35: 50-50

- 25 – 30: 60-70% chance

In summary, it is all just a numbers game.

Just on AMH, for the first IVF cycle, my AMH was 44.4 pmol/l. In 2009 it was 22.72 pmol/l and by 2010 it had dropped to 18.3 pmol/l. To put that in context (the ranges we were given at the time were):

Optimal fertility: 28.6 – 48.5 pmol/l (over 48.5 indicates polycystic ovarian disease (PCOS) or granulosa cell tumours)

Satisfactory fertility: 15.7 – 28.6 pmol/l

Low fertility: 2.2 – 15.7 pmol/l

Very low/undetectable: 0.0 – 2.2 pmol/l

I was now 34. We decided to go with the odds so it was IVF again (this time the long protocol, and it so was). Dr Stats explained that they were used to dealing with very busy people. So much so that they simply tweak the process around their clients' timetables. So, as she told us, a lady in Bahrain would simply phone on day one of her cycle and hey presto the smooth operation that is the Lainsborough would swing into action and plan her meds and trip to London accordingly. It was tailor-made IVF for women who have everything and want results immediately.

But I should have known from that first waiting room experience that the reality was going to be quite different. This was a conveyor belt. A very, very large conveyor belt. And a conveyor belt which required lots of oiling with wads of cash. So we paid our wad and off we went.

Firstly – the Lainsborough is at the arse end of nowhere as far as public transport in London is concerned. The longer I spent there, the more I realised that this was because people who attended it were not exactly your archetypal public transport bods. So, it was fine if you went everywhere by taxi or chauffeur-driven car which a lot of women there seemed to do but for everyone else: add 45 minutes to any trip across London just to get there.

Secondly – timing: arrive for your appointment on time (even if this requires running and arriving as a sweaty stressed mess, again). They won't be on time but if you aren't you will no doubt be shoved further down the queue. Nah, that's rubbish – you will be a long way down the queue anyway so sod it, don't do what I did, just turn up when you feel like it and take a good book. It wasn't until the third scan that I realised the process was: scan (to be fair, usually roughly on time) followed by blood test – anywhere between 45 minutes and 2 hours later. The first time I thought this was just bad luck. The second time I thought maybe they were having a bad day. The third time I asked them what the fuck was going on. To which the response came that the standard process is to have at least 45 minutes between the two. Why? No reason; that's the way it is. Now, medically (from what I can tell) that is bollocks. But more importantly you think they might have mentioned that. So, designed for people who actually have to work to pay for their IVF? I don't think so.

Thirdly – customer service. I was seeing the same two nurses for my blood tests, every other day or so. Did they recognise me – did they hell. Now, maybe these two women were just not very good at remembering faces or names. Or maybe the conveyor belt was so long and so relentless that they didn't notice and didn't care whose arm they were sucking blood out of.

One nurse, phoning with blood test results went one better, "you have excellent AMH, excellent follicle growth and are young (really? Had she read my notes?), so why on earth aren't you pregnant?" Genuinely. She actually asked that question. You know what, given the vast quantities of money (currently standing at £8k) we were paying you, I was kinda hoping (ok, expecting), that is what you, or at least someone there, was going to tell me the answer to that question…

It was also not Jason's favourite place – despite obviously a huge refurbishment and oodles of cash the room in which the men are asked to provide their sample is on a corridor. So, whilst trying to "read" he also had to listen to a conversation between two nurses just outside the door. Not really very helpful. But it did have a nice cubicle in the wall to put the sample in, so at least he didn't have to wander the halls looking vacant and embarrassed trying to find someone to hand his sample to.

It got better.

Collection day came; 15 eggs, all fertilised. They suggested we wait until day 5 (so they can better assess the most viable embryos). By day 5 there were two morulas but no blastocysts, nothing to freeze. Apparently, that's like coming a poor second but it was still good enough to put embryos back in so I was ecstatic. After the transfer procedure it was off across London by tube to get to an acupuncture appointment to "aid implantation and help me relax" except a 45-minute tube ride and a run up the street to get to the appointment on time (queue sweaty mess again) was hardly making relaxation the order of the day. Bear with me, I still hadn't got the hang of the word "relax".

Then the wait began. It actually all felt like it had gone pretty well and then the day before D-day … spotting, maybe that was a good sign? Implantation? Then more that night, more the next day. I'm not sure why I bothered (it's on the list, they need it for their stats) but I did the pregnancy test. Negative. Of course.

The tests, the appointments, the drugs, the stabbing yourself. All a pain in the arse but fine, I can deal with all of that. The mental side, not so much. I hated being bitter but I was finding it so hard to be anything but.

The flood arrived, combined with horrific cramping, as if just to ram it home – you really, really aren't pregnant.

I wanted to hide, make it all go away. No more doctors, no more waiting, no more pain, no more thinking about it, no more false hope. Just stop.

But always, there was the other voice, urging me to do what I always used to think I was good at: fight, push, keep going, do whatever it takes, don't stop until it works. And maybe therein lies the whole problem. If I wasn't such a pushy nightmare maybe I too would be popping out sprogs like there was no tomorrow.

So back we went, once more, to the dreaded waiting rooms, for the follow up appointment. The conclusion, "unfortunately implantation did not occur. There is no explanation for why this happened and hopefully in the next treatment cycle you will do better". Oh I'm sorry, I thought we came here for a scientific view, an understanding of what was going on (or not as the case may be). I didn't realise i) this was all my fault and ii) it was all a question of luck and hope. The bottom line: "it's just a question of running the numbers again" – so pay us more and we'll have another go. They even provided a prescription for the next lot of IVF drugs so we could get right to it. Trying to find the reason why you can't get pregnant, trying to understand what the problem is; most definitely not – just keep throwing money and drugs at it and eventually something might work, it is after all an industry with a single purpose – run the IVF cycle and if it doesn't work, run it again and if that doesn't work, run it again.

6

Looking further afield

"Whatever course you decide upon, there is always someone to tell you that you are wrong. There are always difficulties arising which tempt you to believe that your critics are right. To map out a course of action and follow it to an end requires courage."

Ralph Waldo Emerson

Given the doctors, and allegedly top doctors at that, were so devoid of ability or desire, or both, to find out the reason for infertility we decided to do more of our own research. We took blood tests at home to check for allergies (it turned out I was allergic to cow's milk), did hair tests to check for issues with minerals and metals (it turned out I didn't have enough potassium, chromium, manganese, selenium, vanadium or zinc but did have too much tin) and we started taking far more supplements. We were hardly living the ideal lifestyle so maybe we could solve it by popping a shed load of pills. At least that's what I thought. Jason thought it was a load of nonsense but, no doubt to appease me, agreed to go along with it.

Next, we tried a clinic specialising in miscarriages. Now four years in and Dr Helpful but Critical (so called because he was the first doctor to even come close to trying to find out what the problem was but he also had quite a rude, patronising manner) was the first person to even suggest a thyroid problem.

My thyroid (Thyroid Stimulating Hormone, TSH) was at 4.89 and I had borderline high natural killer cells. According to Dr Helpful but Critical (and, as I now started to read, the research), TSH needs to be 2 or under to have a good chance of getting pregnant. Four years of fertility treatment had passed and not a single doctor or other medical professional had even mentioned the thyroid as a possible issue. I was actually already on levothyroxine (which should have been obvious to all the previous doctors as I put it on every medical assessment form), so, with this further blow to my fast-diminishing faith in the medical profession I started self-medicating and increased the dose.

Dr Helpful but Critical also noted, in the most scathing tones, that I hadn't brought the right documents with me, I clearly hadn't asked the previous doctors the right questions, I didn't even know what was in one of the potions I was still taking from Dr Blunt. He then muttered under his breath about Dr Perfect, that the potion may affect the blood test, relieved me of £1,000 and sent me for blood tests which required 11 vials to be taken.

I went and did the blood tests there and then.

As I got back on the underground to go back to work it turned out that the plaster from the blood test really hadn't really done its job. I could feel something running down my arm inside my suit sleeve. Cautiously I looked down to see drops of blood trickling out from my sleeve, and into my bag. Feeling embarrassed but also thoroughly sick of the whole thing, I looked up. Heavily pregnant woman on one side. New mother with a double buggy on the other. For fuck's sake.

The prescription: get the TSH down, steroids starting at the next ovulation (assuming I could work out when that was, or if it even happened) and vitamin D.

Within three months, the TSH was down to 4.22. Come on.

7

In need of therapy

"When all your world is torn with grief and strife, think yet - when there
seems nothing left to mend, the frail and time-worn fabric of your life, the
golden thread of courage has no end."

Anon (quoted in The Queen's Christmas

Broadcast, 1981)

Therapy had always scared me. I'd never thought I really had any issues
(not real ones anyway) but I still didn't want to be "unpacked". But then I
had started dreaming about suicide and being murdered. And things were
getting worse not better, so off I went. Maybe this was the key?

I trudged across a large park, in the dark with pants street lighting, to a big
Victorian house which seemed to have been split into flats. I rang the bell.
Up the stairs to the top. I could smell the joss sticks before I even got to
the room. The soft lighting. The cushions artfully "scattered". What was

I doing here? I wanted to sort myself out and get pregnant, not enter the twilight zone.

At the end of the first meeting the analytical psychotherapist (Judgmental Therapist as she came to be known) told me, "you are leaking and porous. You need to contain yourself. Get back to a sense of yourself. You are letting everyone into the bedroom (metaphorically speaking) and they should be in the sitting room".   I was on steroids at this point (from Dr Helpful but Critical) which, it seemed, were having a detrimental impact on my mental health. Could I stop them for a month? Apparently, I needed to be able to, "back away from the edge".

There were more gems to follow, "You are emotionally immature. Something, someone has caused that over time. Your dreams show you are a tortured person. You are not far from a nervous breakdown. Gather yourself in, you are leaking everywhere, especially at work (i.e. crying – at least I think that was what she meant and not that she had some amazing prescient knowledge of my incontinence). Intellectually you operate at a high level but emotionally, you are far below, you are not developed".

And there was more: "you have lost your ability to make decisions; to discern for yourself between what the different doctors say. You are unravelling. A bit of you is in freefall. You need to be less judgmental of yourself." It went on, "you have an internal tyrant, which is driving you towards a nervous breakdown. Stop forcing everything. Take a few months off. You don't know how to stop. Say no."

It went on. Apparently, there is "narcissistic damage, you think you have to be perfect, you won't be loved unless you are perfect, that lowers your self-esteem, which is then a vicious circle … you have to be perfect to be loved". Apparently my first real City job did a lot of the damage. That is where I worked 17-hour days, competed to work the hardest, be the best, worked weekends, cancelled holidays etc.

But it wasn't all bad, "you are not psychotic." Oh, thank goodness, that's a relief. And, apparently, "it's only a partial nervous breakdown. If it was a full nervous breakdown then you would be at home in bed, unable to function at all." And, best of all, "you can break the cycle, get back to who you were before."

And then the parts Jason would like: "You need to reignite the feminine (hair, clothes, wax, nails). Read about the Queen of Sheba; there are different sides to being feminine. It can be about cleansing and detoxing. You have too much of the masculine." So it turns out Jason was being helpful and prescient (not rude and annoying as I thought at the time) when he had bought me "How to be Chic and Elegant" following by "What Not to Wear" and "What Not to Wear 2" as Christmas presents three years in a row.

"You can't possibly make a baby because you are not engaged with your husband, either sexually or on an emotional level. It is a masochistic relationship with a narcissistic man, the Oedipus complex but you are fulfilling the daughter role and you need to be in the mother role. You have no concept of appropriate boundaries. It is not normal to want to impress, to not say no to such a huge degree."

"Should you change your name?" I had not changed my surname when we got married. I just never really saw why women should – I have my name, he has his name, I'm not his property or vice versa. Seriously, even my feminist principles were now in play. No, actually, I don't think I am a feminist. I believe in equality. The man never changing his name and the woman always changing her name is not equal.

And on it went, "You need to address who you are. You have low self-esteem (no shit Sherlock and believe it or not this tirade of character "analysis" is not helping hugely). Look at the history of strong, yet feminine women. Don't judge so harshly. Others or yourself. People are not weak because they care about how they look."

So I did look at myself. And I did my homework…

I decided I wanted to return to:

- A strong sense of myself
- Being an individual
- Caring about myself, and others
- Accepting others (not judging them)
- Not being bitter (I was well and truly wallowing in bitterness and pity on a daily basis)
- Being in control
- Living in the now (not dwelling on the past and panicking about the future)
- Trusting my intuition

But my views of "feminine" (if I am brutally honest) were the following:

- Weak
- Stupid
- Not analytical/irrational
- Vacuous
- Incapable of driving (not sure why that was in there but there we go)
- Subservient
- Women do everything; men do what they want

Her advice:

- Know yourself so you can be free
- Know yourself so you have a healthy self-esteem
- There is a good feminine; rejoice in being a woman
- Learn to say no
- Identify bad thoughts – don't speak so fast – consider first
- Boundaries are very important
- Centre yourself each day and check at the end of the day how you did

Judgemental Therapist told me a lot of home truths, and made me think and examine myself, which it turned out I badly needed to do, but it also felt like a battering in and of itself. She had categorised the problem and at least made me feel it was real, too real, but it didn't really unlock the key to what I should do about it. Or maybe I just wasn't ready to do the hard work to make the necessary changes.

The summary seemed to be: slap on some lippy, wear a few more skirts, cut out the crying (so that isn't feminine?) and bob's your uncle you'll be up the duff before you can say "relax".

I started trying to look at what else I might be doing "wrong" which was stopping me getting pregnant. After the great therapy experience I thought something more grounded would be a good bet. Off I went to see a dietician. Apparently, Ribena, Diet Coke and Crunchy Nut Cornflakes (for breakfast and lunch and occasionally supper) is not the optimum diet for baby-making.

So the prescription was reduce your refined sugar intake, take fertility herbs and vitex cassius (whatever the hell that was).

I actually went cold turkey on the sugar. Three days and three very, very long nights. Wow, I thought 17-hour work days made you tired but they were nothing compared to not eating sugar. Apparently after three days, your system gets used to no sugar and you start to "glow" and feel wonderfully re-vitalised. Having tried it, I can tell you, empirically, that is bollocks. But it was a start, to be eating more healthily and thinking about things more holistically.

8

IVF Diary – Going Local

"My dear, in the midst of hate, I found there was, within me, an invincible love. In the midst of tears, I found there was, within me, an invincible smile. In the midst of chaos, I found there was, within me, an invincible calm. I realized, through it all, that…in the midst of winter, I found there was, within me, an invincible summer. And that makes me happy. For it says that no matter how hard the world pushes against me, within me, there's something stronger – something better, pushing right back."

Albert Camus

Just over five years had now passed. A lot of money, heartache, pain and still, nothing.

Feeling increasingly desperate but also like a pinball, we gave up on the London clinics and I looked closer to home. Back to our local fertility clinic. This time straight to Dr Relax.

His advice? You guessed it, "You need to relax. You can't go on doing the same thing and expect a different result."

Until now I never thought there was either anything wrong or any other way to approach work than hard. I had always assumed the only way I had ever achieved anything was by working hard. Therefore, were I to stop working hard, all the achievements would vanish and I would be revealed as the idiot/half-wit I had always feared I was.

So I hadn't worked smart, as advocated by one ex-boyfriend. I hadn't trusted in my own abilities. I hadn't thought that maybe getting to Oxford, 3 As at A level, a scholarship, a job at a global law firm, making partner at 30 might be as a result of anything but hard work. As I was saying, actually a half-wit.

In fact I was so wedded to the Protestant work ethic that by 27 my eyesight had dropped from -7 to -9. In three months. No, that didn't ring alarm bells – it just irritated me, as it meant I had to take some time off work to go to Moorfields Eye Hospital for them to tell me there was nothing wrong with my eyes. I had just strained them so much with working such long hours that my prescription really had changed that fast and no, it wasn't reversible. To assess my eyes the doctor at Moorfields had done that thing where they massively dilate your pupils so you can't see properly for about 2 hours. Did I let that stop me going back to work? Did I hell. I used the walls of the buildings between the hospital and the underground to guide me (literally brushing my hand along as I walked) then squinted and squinted to try and identify the right tube line to get back to…. work. No wonder I thought I was stupid.

For months and months, okay, years, I was finding work increasingly difficult. Being a partner I would sit through endless meetings discussing petty politics: so and so down the corridor is doing this work and we should be doing it; so and so says we have to use this template and we want to use that template. And then my favourite conversations: graduate recruitment – we have selected too many women, "everyone knows that at five years' qualified they will be gone" (read, off to have babies, never to return, or potentially, return but no longer committed to the cause, skiving off to pick children up (no one mentioned that they then usually log back in and work the evenings); the amount of maternity leave is ridiculous and they even get accrued holidays while on maternity leave (to be fair I agree with that one). So, in one of these interminable meetings, I suggested, "well, we could just sterilise all the women". Pause, silence. Several men (and there were only men in the room, apart from me and according to Judgemental Therapist I'm mostly male anyway) were clearly thinking about it...would that work? And then finally embarrassed sighs, "oh, she's just joking".

Anyway, to return to the point at hand, interminable meetings about bollocks, with still a full day's work and a 4 hour commute to fit in.

It was finally at Jason's suggestion and with his support and encouragement: I quit.

So, one big tick for Dr Relax.

Although, as ever, things are never quite that easy. The pressure started with my boss: "you've wrecked me" (he was due to retire, I was supposed to take over his client base). My assistant cried for two hours, "you can't leave me here" followed by "how could you do this to me?"

So the guilt abounded but also a small bit of happiness and hope. All the guilt laden pleadings were lovely in a way (it is always nice to be wanted even if for others' selfish reasons) but that is the point – I wouldn't be staying for me, I would be staying for them and the energy zapping, draining work environment would just carry on.

Dr Relax was right; something fundamental did need to change, I couldn't have it all. I set up my own business. No maternity rights but freedom and control. I had never felt so alive. If I were ever to get pregnant, and it seemed a very remote if, I would deal with the financial/work implications then.

However, Jason did also agree another IVF was possible and, amazingly, our stars had aligned in some way, we had won the postcode lottery - it could be on the NHS this time.

At the initial IVF appointment Jason's sperm had 96% abnormal morphology, i.e. only 4% was good and the World Health Organisation recommended 15%, so it was going to be ICSI. I was now 35, so they put the chance of success at 25-30% and a 15-20% twin pregnancy rate if two embryos were transferred.

The day after the appointment Jason said the sperm test results had been an epiphany moment for him and that he had been in denial for the last five years; he hadn't wanted anything to be wrong so in his mind there had been nothing wrong. Simple as that. How I wished I had that much control over my thought processes. Finally, it seemed we were on the same page.

13 September. Day 1 of the IVF cycle. Or more correctly, day 1 of the cycle before the IVF cycle. Spoke to Judith and she said she would organise everything and not to worry. But it did worry me. It worried me that she was masquerading as a nurse. Was she a nurse or a secretary?

I didn't know what I felt. A little bit dead really and tired, so very tired of it all. And this period is a real nightmare, it feels like the Dyson is on in full suction mode: went to sleep trying to ignore the pain. Huge clots – why would anyone in their right mind volunteer to be a woman? As Jason is always saying, never trust anything that bleeds for a week a month and doesn't die.

14 September. Had counselling this morning. Lovely house in the Home Counties, a specialist in fertility counselling. Apparently, that is now a thing. Therefore, eminently able to help.

After an hour, her advice? You just need to get pregnant and then all this will go away. No shit Sherlock. I had that one figured out (although to be fair I was starting to wonder if my new crazy was going to be permanent so, I concede, it is helpful to know that was not the case).

I spent most of the hour talking about Jason, his drinking and denial; my nagging and guilt at having been a witch for the last 5 years. We also talked a little bit about how I see this as my failure – and that I had it coming to me for all the good things I've had in life. She seemed horrified when I told her the previous counsellor had said I had lost all touch with my feminine side. So, I guess that is a plus.

In fact, I still feel okay which is good; well actually just tired (partly physical because I have been up at 5 a.m. to go to some stupid breakfast meeting which made me late for the counselling which kind of sums up the whole problem – there I went again putting work first). That'll teach me. You would have thought it would have sunk in by now. By the afternoon I had said no to any future breakfast "networking" events; maybe was I learning? Also had acupuncture with a new acupuncturist (Roger) closer to home and even managed not to cry – result. He recommended a local herbalist, Magda. I often wonder if they are all getting a cut from each other…

15 September. Not a bad day. Busy with work and admin so not really thinking about things. Got upset about receiving a brochure for kids' stuff in the post but really just because it all feels so very far away. Getting pregnant and having kids just seems to be something that happens to other people.

16 September. Pretty good day – busy with things so feeling pretty positive about life generally. Also went to see the new herbalist, Magda, who seemed to know her stuff and wants me to bring her all the pills and supplements I am on so she can do a full assessment.

17 September. Went to pick up sheep from Dorset which took all day but kind of showed me quite how far I have come from spending all day in the office arguing politics, tending to the emotional needs of others, working. But overall, this sort of day – out in the real world and not working makes me feel so lucky. Looks like Jason has secured the move at work he wants which is fantastic news – I hope that will help him look forward and bring the challenge and enjoyment (to a degree) back to work for him which seems to have been missing for so long.

19 September. Just so tired. Trying not to be down. Not doing very well at that. Just feel tired of everything – back to feeling that pregnancy is something that happens to other people. Saw Paula today (about 7 months pregnant); Andrea and Claire talking about their kids – which of course they would and should. I'm not even at the stage of thinking this round won't work – just all seems so distant; the thought of being pregnant let alone having children just seems like it's something from another lifetime – not mine, it's not real. Not here, not now. Tired of talking about it – I think Jason must be bored to death of it. Please, someone, change the record.

20 September. Not a bad day – just busy with work. It is incredible how the Protestant work ethic can make you happier (or at least less depressed) by taking your mind off things. Anyway, tonight was the long-awaited call with Dr Sami David – author of The Fertility Plan. He of the Stuck/Pale/Tired/Dry/Waterlogged way of thinking but more importantly, the first doctor in New York to undertake a successful IVF treatment and seemingly the first to disown the IVF industry and instead, shock, horror, try to find out why people can't get pregnant. Now that is innovation or at least a new concept… Jason came home early and over a pretty bad mobile phone line to New York we were asked more questions that at any other appointment in the last five years. In fact, make that the last five years' worth of appointments altogether. And that, we discovered half-way through was without (or maybe because of a lack of) the 60 pages of our medical records I had lovingly spent hours scanning to him over a month ago. We were impressed (not by the admin screw up; but by the advice). I felt an inkling of hope again and not just because it was yet another new avenue, new things to do and check, but real new hope that maybe this time we might find the key to it all. There has been a honeymoon period with every doctor we have seen – the only distinguishing feature is how fast our hope and their seeming competence crashes and burns - so we'll see but so far it is looking good.

The other thing that made it full of hope was that since his epiphany, this was us actually doing something together. Dr David's advice was that I need 4 blood tests, a culture of cervical mucus and a post coital test but that it looks like my prolactin is elevated, and that with high TSH as well it looks like a luteal phase deficiency. He said not to use the embryos we have stored until they worked out what was going on and that vitamins shouldn't be necessary if you have a good diet but if you don't then 1 milligram of folic acid, omega 3 and vitamin D plus food high in zinc. Jason only needs a semen analysis and to stop roasting his testicles in boiling hot baths (in fact, rather than lowering the temperature of the bath, it is better to forget them altogether and just shower) and finishing them off by having his phone in his front pocket but still, at least there were some questions for him and some participation. Dr David did actually also say to limit alcohol intake to 3 units at any one time but I'm not sure that sunk in.

21 September. Spent the day, in and around work, trying to find someone, anyone who would do a post coital test or blood tests (any test in fact) without a letter of referral. It would appear being willing to give up your own blood is not enough, not even if you are paying for it.   Some random punter with the initials DR in front of their name has to approve it. What is the fear – that people max out on tests – provided you're paying what does it matter? And on the post coital test it was as if I had asked for the national debt to be worked out on an abacus. Did I not know that this was old science? The disdain. My GP (stand-in) hadn't even heard of one but seemed grateful for the whistle-stop tour of infertility medicine. The fertility clinic won't do it; the NHS don't know what it is; the private hospital who might do it never returned my calls; the internet, for once, was equally useless.   Apparently, it has been rendered completely unnecessary by the new innovations in IVF. Yup. Knew that. Just find me somewhere that does the fucking test. Reminded me of Dr Helpful but Critical who literally laughed in my face when I asked for a prolactin test. Oh wait, let's see, how does this work again? I pay you extortionate sums of money. I ask for particular tests. You say no – with a laugh and a sneer.

22 September. Result – managed to persuade The Doctors Laboratory that despite it being old science, despite there being strict requirements about the timing (of sex – or as the lady rather sweetly and utterly naively referred to it – making love), despite forcing them to go to the inconvenience of getting a doctor in specially and despite the cost at over £300 – YES – for my mad sins, I did want a post coital test. How relative things become – I was elated to find someone willing to stick yet another contraption up me and scrap out some goo; and pay them handsomely for the pleasure. Also managed to get the prolactin and TSH tests booked. I then asked for the results to be sent to me. No. No, it is not possible for your own blood and cervical culture test results to be sent to you. Not without the written consent of your doctor. I started pointing out that it was my blood and my cervical mucus but realised I was on a sticky wicket (sorry, couldn't resist), so for once, stopped.   Am amazed at how more peaceful and less angry I feel. Before I would have railed, become indignant in that incredibly pompous lawyerly way; instead I managed (almost gracefully) to accept what they were saying and made a note to get the consent.

23 September. The IVF drugs arrived today – smaller box and more tightly packed than before - including some vaginal gel (hmmm did I really ask for that or is that what constitutes an IVF freebie?). A nice man delivered them – he undid the box to show me which ones to put in the fridge. Strange the jobs some people have.   Feeling okay about it – except that the needles look much bigger and more medical somehow. Which is clearly ridiculous. Still doesn't feel very real at the moment.

Then out of nowhere got a one line email from Dr David's secretary/assistant saying elevated prolactin level take Bromocriptine. Just like that. Feels great – at last another step to actually finding out what is wrong and then, God forbid, fixing it.   Have decided I am too judgmental about doctors. The problem is I assume that they are logical and scientific when in fact it is an art like everything else. So when I assume they will identify the problem and then apply the appropriate fix; it would appear that instead, they have their own views, thoughts, preconceptions, prejudices and philosophies about the problem and therefore the solution.

25 September. Ovulation test – negative. Started the day with a session with Patricia, the therapist/counsellor assigned by the clinic. I really don't get these people. I arrived, on time; she was late. "How is the cycle going now that you are half-way through?" "I haven't actually started taking the drugs but it is fine thanks". She was actually sitting there with my file. She was late anyway – why not take a minute to see where I actually was in the treatment cycle. Mind you at least she recognised me – which is more than can be said for the staff at the Lainsborough.

So we talked – well I talked and she said the odd thing. I talked about Jason and how I thought he had been so much better since his epiphany and yet when he lists the things "wrong that need to be fixed" there is my thyroid and now prolactin level. His semen analysis seems strangely missing from the list. I hadn't mentioned it to him at the time – there seemed little point. But on reflection, despite the alleged epiphany, his denial still seems pretty much intact – her words not mine. She then asked how I felt about the fact that he didn't really seem to be supporting me. I don't know. Is it pure frustration; anger; disappointment? Or is it even understanding? I think the thing that has bothered me most about all this infertility stuff and Jason is really the surprise – I thought we were incredibly strong, I thought I knew him and how he thought about things. I love him so much and I had figured he felt the same way and yet over this, over something so difficult, we just don't seem to meet in the middle.

And what does that mean – that the love I thought was there is illusory? That actually for all our "communication" we aren't really getting through to each other? We are just talking at each other but neither of us is listening? Why is it that even with a sperm test as bad as it was, even after 5 years of trying, even after all the operations I've had and drugs I've taken, even after one of the top doctors in the US says he may need to see a specialist and not to have more than three units a night; the binge drinking continues, the sense (albeit not as bad as before) that this is just my problem pervades – it is something I (not we) want; it is something I nag about; it is my agenda, not his? I don't understand. He scoffs when I say maybe he is an alcoholic – he himself admitted that he wants to drink all the time (to escape his thoughts and mind; to relax).

So, in summary the feedback from the counsellor was that I am alone, have a husband in denial, and no one else to turn to. But then she followed up, once again, with, "not to worry, if you get pregnant all this will just go away and if you don't then you should both see me for couple counselling as you're going to need it." Wow, where do they find these people?

From there I went to Sarah and Tony's to be met at the door by John (Sarah's brother) and his three week old son. There must have been 20 kids there of varying ages. And virtually every parent moaning about their lot. I don't understand that – no doubt because I don't have children, but are they really that annoying that it is a relief when someone else offers to have them for just a few short hours? Going on the market research to date of friends and neighbours that does appear to be the case. Sat with

Tom (Sarah's eldest and my godson) for quite a while who is just gorgeous – but it does remind me of what I don't have.

Card got rejected at petrol station on the way home – no money left in my account the nice man informed me. Miraculously I managed to remember the number for my emergency credit card. IVF costs really were taking their toll.

26 September. Ovulation test – negative. Phoned the bank and realised the petrol station man was right – there is simply no money left. We have burnt right through our overdraft.

Jason is away at a university reunion. No call and no text.

Which means one of two things, he is so drunk he forgot or, he has lost his phone (again), or possibly both. Why am I so judgmental? No seriously – where does that come from? Fighting with myself all morning – I should be understanding; he deserves time off; a good time. But this is just fucking ground hog day. And I am tired, so very tired of it. Maybe there is something more serious going on – I get that he doesn't want to be told what to do, no one likes to be told what to do, I get that he likes to drink, I get that that is the social world in which he lives, I get that he liked being Mr Perfect (he, originally, of the perfect sperm), I even get that he may have more of a macho approach to these things than I had previously thought. But why is his denial so pervasive?

It is still me pushing – pushing to go on the call with the US doctor, booking the sperm test, pushing him to come to counselling (which he doesn't), pushing him to take days off to do the IVF, pushing the vitamins, pushing the prolactin research. Nothing (or virtually nothing) is volunteered or offered. Do we just work in different ways at different speeds or do we just want different things? Is it that unless I believe he is actually on board my body will not play ball?

Maybe it is just that he is so much more vulnerable than I had ever realised. How can I not have known that? How much more don't I know? How blind and self-absorbed have I been (and for so long now)?

So here I am again, waiting for him to come home, hung over and tired. No doubt expecting me to explode. Done that already – just broke another vacuum cleaner. It was weird this time – I actually decided I wanted to hit it – so it's getting worse I guess, because this wasn't a heat of the moment but more premeditated. Shit. Maybe I'm just not fit to be a mother. Have thought of another reason why this should never be published – because it is so fucking dull. I'm bored by it and it is about my life. What the hell would anyone else think?

Jason eventually came home, about 2 p.m. It was worse than I thought in some ways – he really had gone for broke this time. When he finally woke up from yet another big night out, he found a receipt in his wallet, with the time of 03.21, for £500 from his favourite kebab shop. He thinks, but is not entirely sure, that he wanted, no, insisted, that he pay for kebabs for every customer for the rest of the night. Oh no, not just his mates, every single person who might fall into the kebab shop that night. Not knowing what the cost might be it appears he plucked a figure out of the air and that happened to be £500.

Aside from being the most gratuitous waste of money (putting the cost of his reunion dinner at approaching £1,000) and the last thing we need right now, it also makes me sad. Tired. Let down. Quietly angry. But mostly sad. So he stood in the kitchen and explained how he wasn't entirely sure how much he had had to drink because he had been so drunk, he couldn't remember but let's face it, it was a long, long way from the three units Dr David had cautioned about only a few days earlier. He could remember the bar before dinner, six glasses with dinner and then it was on from there.

So I sat and cried; well it was more pathetic than that, sobbed really. Here we go again - how fucking tedious is this?

"Do you believe what any doctor says?"

"What does go on in your head?"

"Why are you in denial?"

"Why do you still not do anything proactively?"

The answers?

He doesn't really know. He says he loves me with all his heart and soul. I believe that. He doesn't want anything to be wrong – he wants it to all be okay. Which I guess is the point of denial - self-protection. He does want children. I believe that too. He doesn't think he has a drink problem. He doesn't want to do IVF – not even the cycle we are locked into now. He doesn't want to need to do IVF. He is angry at the doctors and how they haven't asked the right questions – any real questions in fact (Dr David and Dr Helpful but Critical aside) – but have just pushed the party line of IVF.

Had another appointment with Magda. Took the ridiculous stash of supplements we are on – there were so many they filled a whole supermarket bag for life. She was horrified. Probably rightly so; but then when you have so much advice coming at you from so many angles it's hard to know who to believe so you just keep following it all. In Magda's view, I'm stagnant and closed off. Awesome. Oh, and there's too much yearning; and I need a holiday. I could have told her that. My static (i.e. working) lifestyle means there is not enough movement around the uterus so nothing will implant. So, it appears, my system needs a shove (technical term apparently…). A quick six weeks (weirdly at a later appointment it then seemed that three to four months were actually required) on her magic formula and everything will fall into place, just like that. Oh, and I need to go and see a cranial osteopath, weirdly there was one she could recommend… She did also recommend using fertility friend for my charts, which were free, so thankfully it wasn't all about the fertility money tree.

28 September. Positive ovulation test. Yippee. Strange as well that now I am not doing temperature charts and the fertility monitor, I am paying more attention to my body again. So have noticed the signs – mucus, "wet" when I wipe my bottom having peed, tender breasts. This is all so gross. So spoke to the lady in Andrology Solutions. Yes, I do know that a post coital test is unusual and something they haven't done for years but yes I do still want it. She promises to ring back about the timings.

29 September. Today is the day for the post coital test – having had a positive ovulation test yesterday morning means a post coital test at 5 p.m. today which means sex at 5 a.m. The alarm went and off we went (so to speak). No bath, just a minimal shower and let's see whether any sperm are left alive or if my amazing immune system has killed them all off.

The gynaecologist was an hour late (so sex could have been at 6 a.m. but anyway), she came in and performed the test that no one wants to do anymore. Did I know no one does this test anymore? No, really, I hadn't heard that – but please do tell…

It hurt a little (the ignominy of lying with your knees up, legs apart, speculum inserted to keep your vaginal walls apart aside), just the scrapping and then when she couldn't get the mucus off the vaginal wall, the suction effect and nick which drew blood (for which she apologised, so that's ok then). In fact, when I thanked her, she responded that it had been a pleasure – really?! English politeness really does go too far at times. In fact the doctor who arranged the appointment was so effusive I couldn't tell if she was just being nice because she felt sorry for me or pleased to be doing an "unusual" test.

Walking down Wigmore Street, thinking about recent moodiness and anger, it seems that I have taken a few steps back – back to feeling let down, angry, aggressive. Why? How much is tied up with my competitive nature? That I have to win; that life is a race at the end of which we will all be measured. There are always those who seem able to forgive, I don't know why but I often think about that boy who was murdered in a bakery awhile back and his mother said how sorry she felt for the boy who did it and that she had forgiven him. I have never understood that mentality and yet surely it is the way forward – the only way forward if you are to live without bitterness, anger and regret.

Felicity whose new-born died of COTS, said that she cannot be angry because there is nothing and no one to be angry at. There is no one and nothing for me to be angry at and yet for most of the last five years I have been so very, very angry that I have been violent and hurt physical things as well as emotionally lashing out at those I love the most in the world.

So what I need to do (selfishly if you like) is get back to the mentality of forgiveness and understanding. Jason has his own reasons for doing and saying things. Being angry, upset, let down, disappointed won't help me or him. Moving beyond that will.

I am reading Teach Us To Sit Still by Tim Parks. A very good book; it makes me wonder how much of it is true for me? Does my back ache, spine have a T5 twist and left leg no feeling because I have forced everything for so much of my life? Am I not now reaping the seeds I sowed from an early age? Push, push your body – the harder you push the better and more it will respond. Until now I had fundamentally believed it was good to push your body – why else would it feel so good?

At an instinctive level, I feel deeply that my infertility is my fault. My entire life, for what I thought were the very best reasons, I have striven, mind and body to produce the very best that I can. In sport, I have cajoled, forced and in the case of my knees, literally worn out my body in an attempt to get fit for the pitch (before all this I used to play a lot of sport). At the same time, at work, I have literally forced my eyes open, my mind to stay alert for longer and longer hours. All-nighters and what actually takes a far worse toll, the endless late nights, early mornings, weekends and 4-5 hours' sleep a night. Even when my eyesight was failing me I didn't heed the warnings.

Why have I pushed so hard? Was it because I stumbled so badly (physically and academically) at a young age? Was it the Protestant work ethic so engrained by family and school? Hard work and effort are rewarded. Was it hereditary? Is it insecurity, a lack of confidence and therefore a need to constantly prove myself – to myself and others? Is it because of a belief that the things that I saw as "achievements" arose from good luck or hard work alone – not ability. All of those?

30 September. The last day before the drugs start.

1 October. Took first Provera pill. Saw Judith at the fertility clinic. She is a nice lady but I still can't tell if she is a PA or nurse and if the former why on earth is she giving lessons on injecting etc. She seems to be a voyeur, it is almost like she is relishing in the drama and pain of it all. To top it all, her summary: "as this is your third time round you probably don't have much hope". No, thanks for that, you are absolutely right.

The advice from the clinic, which no one else had suggested before, was to drink milk during the IVF cycle. I hate milk but throw some chocolate in and I can just about manage it, so our daily hot chocolate binge began.

2 October. Nothing much to report – second day of Provera and booked Fertility Show for November. That should be a fun day. But hopefully informative…   Jason has agreed to come but as ever there is the undercurrent that I am pushing and he has agreed but it is certainly not something he wants to do. Too tired of it to make an issue out of it.

3 October. Injections started today – funny how it takes you back. Not too bad but already feeling reticent about pushing a needle into myself. If it is like this now wait till we get onto the Gonal F.

4 October. Off to see Dr Relax today. He was okay – I actually ended up feeling sorry for him as he sweated away. Not sure if it is just his way but he does seem to take the negative/realism approach very seriously. Is it really necessary to tell me at the beginning of a cycle that this is the last chance saloon – so there is a one in three chance this could work but once this cycle is done, it is downhill from here. Oh and prolactin – forget it, being over the range isn't really being over the range….apparently he doesn't even take notice of it until it is into four figures…an over the range result can come about just from having an injection. So, the range is not there for a reason? The range is wrong? So no Bromocriptine for me. I didn't push it but felt overwhelmingly depressed as he sat with his empty private prescription pad in front of him – once again batting away concerns/requests for help with a dismissive patronising smile. Fuck you quite frankly. One of the leading doctors in the States is prescribing it but no, that's not good enough for you – you who openly acknowledge that the science of infertility has barely moved on since the 1950s. Well you know what, will it kill me or even harm me to have it? The air just seems heavy with his words from before – "you need to start thinking about the alternatives". Well you know what, I'm so not done yet and my darling husband has already said he wouldn't countenance adoption; so where does that leave me? Fuck it and fuck you.

5 October. Cancelled joint counselling session. No, I don't want to re-book – this process is depressing enough without having a counsellor who can't remember my name, where I am in my treatment and just repeats like an automaton: "and how does that make you feel?" To be fair, she has another stock phrase, "it is hard, very hard." Oh, and occasionally, "Everyone going through what you are going through finds it that way". The down-beat approach seems to be the in-thing here; but then I moaned about the doctors in London with their hope-filled bags of hot air. Who knows.

6 October. Michael's wife's funeral. Just sat and cried the whole way through – possibly made worse by the drugs and hormones but also just so desperately sad. Actually decided before I went that something needs to change and just thinking how self-consumed I've been for the last 5 years. So after this cycle (on the assumption it doesn't work) Jason will be in charge. I know I will find that very hard and I'm guessing there will be a lot of "let's just have loads of sex, alcohol and see how it goes" but then five years of pushing, shoving, top doctors and potions and injections haven't got us anywhere so why not? He seems ok with the idea – we'll see.

7 October. Fertility Show tickets arrived. Wahoo there's something to look forward to.

8 October. Long drive up to Norfolk. Not helped by Jason putting in the wrong postcode so we went the wrong way and to the wrong place but I actually managed to not be a complete witch about it – quite some achievement.

9 October. David and Ziva's wedding day. Really beautiful ceremony; only 20 guests. The happy couple were all over each other like a hot rash. Made me wonder what happened to all that – when did sex become such a chore, with such negative connotations? But then the pain and blood really don't help. Really hard to inject today – just couldn't make my hand stab myself and then got ridiculous when I missed and stabbed my finger so had to start all over again. What has making babies come to?

10 October. Long drive back from Norfolk, interspersed with lunch at Jason mother's. She asked how it was going or whether we had given up, so slightly embarrassing moment when I said we were currently doing an IVF cycle and she asked what that was. I thought she read the Daily Mail surely that has at least one IVF miracle per week? I looked to Jason; he muttered something about test tubes. She thinks it is all me – nothing could possibly be wrong with her perfect boy – so she is in good company with the very well-paid specialists but to be fair she hasn't hassled or harried me about the whole thing and for that, I will be eternally grateful.

11 October. Injection hurt going in this morning but no blood so hopefully have escaped another bruise. Had vague thought that I might be pregnant (chance would be a fine thing) as period still hasn't arrived but only day 29 so guess it will be tomorrow.

12 October. Acupuncture. Needles, needles.

13 October. It's all about definitions. No, Judith I did not "wake up bleeding" but I did start bleeding before 1 p.m. Approximately 12.30 to be precise. So in my book that makes this day 1. But as with all fertility doctors – who the fuck knows. So I spoke to Judith to book a day 4 blood test after which the "uppers" start. Now that should mean Saturday but oh no, no one takes blood on a Saturday so that means it has to be Monday. Which is day 6. Had shiatsu massage – weird and expensive but then that seems to be my taste (when it comes to fertility treatment anyway).

16 and 17 October. Had people to stay for Saturday night and Sunday lunch. It was nice to see people but felt absolutely exhausted. What is wrong with me? I used to be able to do 2 all-nighters in a row without even batting an eyelid. Ridiculous.

18 October. Absolutely foul mood and just can't shake it. Best to stay away from people. Just feel utter despair. Am betting this cycle won't work and then where are we – back at fucking square one after 5 very long years. What is the fucking point? Had blood test and blood pressure taken. Just feel so arsey. Trying not to be rude but it is an uphill battle. Phoned by the all-knowing Judith who told me to start the Gonal F tomorrow. So there is something to look forward to after all.

19 October. Had all my hair cut off (well, okay, just very short). Strange – I guess it was a big decision but just said do it. Feels much better- let's see how long that lasts.

20 October. Started bleeding – assume it is just a hangover from my period. Sounds awful but just not sure I am that bothered anymore.

21 October. Still bleeding – apparently nothing to worry about just the hormones sorting themselves out. Hmm. How great it is to be a woman. Just not seeing how this is going to work. All I can see is Dr Relax at the "post event" appointment talking about "other options" and the need to consider them and then Jason and I having a row because he won't adopt. Brilliant.

22 October. Went to see Sophie and Rachel. So lots of children. Sophie helpfully pointed out that I have my priorities all wrong and work too hard… Friends… Here's hoping I haven't left it too late.

23 and 24 October. Amazing weekend where I actually did very little. Wow – this must be how other people live. Saw Jason's mum who noted that someone had said to her lawyers don't have children or can't get pregnant because they are too busy. Is there anyone else who wants to have a pop?

25 October. First scan today. It appears that they make everyone arrive at the same time, change into gowns and bath robes and sit in the same room. I couldn't decide if knickers were on or off – went with off which luckily was right. One girl turned up with her boyfriend/husband who asked everyone in the waiting room if they minded him being there. How sweet is that? Also, I know Jason is very busy at work and this is an important time for him but it just made me realise how some blokes approach it and surely that can only help – imagine that, doing the process together. Instead, when Jason came home and I said that I still didn't know what days the collection and transfer were going to be he tutted and rolled his eyes in irritation. It wasn't anger and I wasn't angry at him – just not sure I have the energy anymore to be angry and I do understand but it would still be nice not to feel, once a fucking gain that it is me pushing, me forcing him through a process and me messing with his meeting calendar for the next few weeks. But that is the reality. I am the one messing with it. Yes, he is loads better on the alcohol front but this is clearly still something I am doing; not both of us. That has come out all wrong and I don't actually feel that bothered or angry anymore but I guess I just thought how nice it would be if Jason was there with me. It was also just weird sitting in a room of women all wanting the same thing, all studiously ignoring each other, all – bar one, there without their husbands/boyfriends/girlfriends. Reminded me of broody hens, sitting, waiting for days on end not knowing if there is going to be anything worth talking about at the end of the process or just a rotten egg. Based on current odds it would seem that only two out of the eight of us will succeed this time. Which brings us back to Dr Relax's question – what happens if this doesn't work? But on the statistics front, there seem to be about 7 follicles each side, all about 10-12 mm; which is good.

26 October. Now bleeding from my bottom. That really can't be right. So decided it was time to do those stool tests which I was going to put off until after the IVF. I have a feeling it may just be piles – how embarrassing is that? Then the lights went out at 9 am and I remembered that the power was going off for a day for maintenance. So now sitting at

Mum and Dad's trying to get their broadband to work so I can do some actual work. Starting to feel quite bloated.

27 October. Second scan this morning – the place seems to be in disarray but there was one more follicle (or seemed to be – Dr Relax said there were 8 on the left and 7 on the right and then couldn't find it again – who knows…). But they are growing and that seems a good number so still in the game. Two husbands and someone's mother and various children were there this time. I just think bringing children to a fertility clinic is incredibly insensitive. OK there maybe the odd occasion when you really can't find childcare and I get it that secondary infertility can be as bad but honestly – is that really the right thing to do? Anyway. Collection now seems set for Monday or Tuesday so phoned Jason. He was fine but then said, "I have to go; got things to do." I'm sure he does and I know he's very busy but once again it is starting to feel very lonely. He says things take a while to sink in with him – fine – but this is glacial. I'll be at the menopause before he has even accepted there is a problem getting pregnant.

Got an email from Dr David about our tests. The sperm analysis appears to be within normal parameters although there were slightly increased levels of cytoplasmic droplets which, it seems, can lead to DNA damage and can indicate sperm production which occurs in high heat environments – so, as the awesome Dr David had already advised, get the bath temperature down and the mobile in the back pocket. On my side, with apologies for the grossness, the mucus isn't good enough quality for the sperm to be able to swim properly (instead of 5-10/hpf (whatever that means) I was at 1/hpf and instead of at least 30% motility, I was at 25%. The fix – it feels like we are back where we started: guaifenesin (i.e. cough medicine).

28 October. Up to London today to see Rosemary. I really like her but always feel a bit nervous which is ridiculous. We talked a bit about fertility treatments and her daughter. Having my own family just seems so very, very far away.

29 October. Last scan. I was last this time. So sat there watching the others and in my head wishing them luck. The woman in the first couple looked really sad – hard to know if she is just down about the whole thing or if it is not going that well. Dr Relax said there were 18 eggs although I had the impression he was making up the last one… oh well.

Had a debate with Dr Relax and Judith about the amount of Gonal F I had left – he said I couldn't take it and to bring it back in. Then she said I could… which was very nice of her. Which one is the doctor?

30 and 31 October. Collection was going to be Tuesday but was changed to Monday at the last minute so desperately trying to get work done. Jason seems to have calmed down on the days off thing which is a relief.

Friends to stay – one lot with their two kids. We were all in the kitchen and Abbie started crying – just so sad – sounds like the depression has been pretty bad and now she is on her own in the house, and working from home – not surprised she is going nuts. Had a good chat about how shit things can be – turns out she was jealous of Jason and me thinking we had it all. So I described some of the incidents from the last five years which showed it had been less than pretty. I think that helped her feel better.

1 November. Collection Day. So up at 6.30 am – drank a pint of water as required. We got to the clinic in good time – they were very efficient. Weird that I was only sedated and yet felt so out of it. They collected 14 eggs. Got home and slept till about 4 pm.

2 November. A report out today shows that women who are stressed have better chances with IVF. Aside from thinking the study is bullshit it's ironic that once I am finally getting to a more relaxed place it turns out I should be stressed. Fucking typical. Oh just stop with the woe is me bollocks. Anyway back to the actual point at hand. They collected 14 eggs. Of which 10 fertilised, using ICSI. So they will watch them and grade them on Thursday and then we make a decision about what goes back in and, if there are any others, what is frozen. We'll see.

Still feels painful but can't tell if that is the operation or the constipation. Or just both. Fairly relaxed day but every now and again I catch myself clenching my jaw. Maybe I am far more uptight about this than I realise. Booked a weekend trip to France for the weekend after next. Not sure if that is a good or bad idea.

3 November. Feel weird today. I think it is probably the constipation. Except it isn't really just that but this massive tightness in my chest – like something huge is stuck there and won't move. Is that just back-up effect from constipation (I remember the first IVF was horrendous on that front) or is it fear or worry? Who knows. I wish I could shake the negative

73

feeling but it just seems to be there, hanging over me. An email from Polly today, she gave birth last night to a son, Tod. Apparently only took 7 hours and she only needed gas and air. I am pleased for her. Of course I am, she is a lovely person and thoroughly deserves to be happy. It's just that it rams it all home AGAIN. I had hoped I had moved on from feeling like that but it seems not. Not that I am feeling anywhere near as angry as I was – I don't have the energy for that. So, tomorrow is transfer day – well, hopefully is transfer day – we have to see how they have developed first. So fingers crossed. Please let my mood become more upbeat. Please.

4 November. Transfer day. Two good ones to go back (8-cell good and 8-cell fair) and three to freeze which is brilliant – the best results yet. The rest go to research.

Wet myself almost every day. And that was when I was staying in bed. So if incontinence is a sign of pregnancy I'm there already.

13 November. Going to France today. Did debate about whether that was a good idea but even Zita West says you should have a weekend away so why not? I bumped into the door handle when carrying the bag down the corridor – the usual sign that my period is coming. Surely not. If things are going to go wrong I kinda thought it would be closer to Thursday. Went to Le Buffet. Nice meal – Jason criticised me for judging him about his drinking when I hadn't even opened my mouth. I did decide if it went to two liqueurs then I was out of there (that on top of the two beers at lunch, the Kir Royale and most of the bottle of wine and the port). Yup there I go judging again. But fucking hell. Feel edgy – can't quite put my finger on it, other than of course the looming Pregnancy Test on Thursday.

14 November. Woke up fine but feeling edgy. Had breakfast. Back to the room to collect our bags. Went to the loo. There it was. Brown mess. My period. The tears just started. Cried with Jason for a bit and then got into the car. Realised after 20 minutes that we had the wrong time for the boat and actually had 30 minutes less time than we thought. Dad started racing for the motorway. Made it in time. Loo stop and by now it is bright red and clots and just unstoppable. Texted Magda – who suggested immediate bed rest and that she would make up some slippery foetus mixture. Insanely, I figured that was a good thing. Also, moxa every hour on the hour.

Magda also explained that there are three reasons why IVF or indeed any pregnancy fails: i) there is something chromosomally wrong so the body rejects the embryo; ii) it fails to implant for some reason; iii) the timing is out (apparently quite frequently the case with IVF in the UK) and therefore you get your period – the body gets to the allotted day and the hormones which dictate it is period time are simply too strong.

She is nice and trying to be supportive but the underlying message is clear – we are now in hurl and hope territory. Again.

Finally got home and straight to bed – now big lumpy clots. Mucus. Blood. Everywhere. Jason picked up the mixture. He seems to think everything will be ok. I, however, think it is all over. There is just too much blood for it not to be.

I just want to cut out my fucking useless uterus. Do they do transplants?

15 November. There is still blood everywhere – it ran down my legs when I went to acupuncture, through my trousers – blood and clots. Disgusting. Roger kindly agrees to do a treatment – a miscarriage prevention treatment but again the message is clear. It may work but it is pretty unlikely. Amid the tears I told him not to worry it wasn't like I was going to hold him to it. My hope pretty much vanished at 9.45 yesterday morning. Phoned the clinic – the nurse number was just voicemail so left a message. To be fair I just said I had been bleeding since yesterday, I assumed I should still go ahead with the test (there are their stats to consider after all) on Thursday and they could call me back if they wanted. The phone didn't ring.   Maybe I should have actually asked for them to call back but what are they going to say? You've just fucked our stats, please don't darken our door again

It was Mark and Alan's wedding today. I didn't go which I feel extremely bad about as I know how crap it is to have people not turning up but it would be hard with so much blood and when I am supposed to be lying down all day.

So I lay and read, bled on the bed (it went through to the mattress), burnt the sheets (with the Moxa), cried, thought a lot, cried some more, felt angry and then just felt dead. I'm just not sure I've got much left. Jason went to the wedding. He seemed so happy – whistling and singing to himself in the kitchen. Is that a defence mechanism? Does he really think it will be ok? Does he just not think about it? I just hope he comes back at a reasonable time – please, please don't let him get drunk and stay out. I just don't think I could bear it.

So what now? Curl up and die. Hide. Give up? I don't know anymore. I really thought I was getting somewhere. Despite my negativity I really thought I was in such a better place that this might be it this time. Did I not eat well enough? I know I could have eaten better – too much sugar and chocolate. Did I do something else wrong? Was I not positive enough? Did I not visualise properly/enough? How the fuck can it be this hard?

Searching the internet for IVF, blood and mucus (Magda asked if there was mucus so I'm guessing that is a bad sign), I found the Pregnancy Miracle. Is it? Can it be? Fuck it – bought a copy to download. Printing all 276 pages of it now.

Jason is home at 11pm – following a nightmare journey through the fog. Just so glad to see him.

16 November. Just wondering what the fucking point is – five years is a long time, that's 60 periods, 60 months of it not working. Why should anything be different from here? Started reading Pregnancy Miracle – got about half way through and to be fair it is helpful but honestly, I just can't see how you can put it all into practice and still have a normal life or is that the point – in order to get pregnant you need to do what I have done the last two months (just focussed on the IVF cycle) and literally do nothing else? If I can't see that working does that mean I'm not that committed and therefore don't deserve to be/won't ever get pregnant?

77

Spoke to Jason about it and started crying. Finally, he explained the plan for the next 9 months – a rules basis with rewards and points. Sounds good; he really has thought this through and finally, finally it seems like he is engaged. It is our problem now, not just mine. At fucking last.

17 November. Killed off the new vac today – I was doing really well when I couldn't get the bits back together – even spotted that I was getting stressed and started deep breathing and then just lost it and hurled it down the corridor, smashing it to pieces. Took extra Gonal F back to the clinic plus a present for Judith and Dr Relax. I bought him Man's Search for Meaning by Viktor Frankl, an incredible book about the Holocaust but also, in a more general way, the desperation caused by uncertainty. Judith phoned and said she assumed everything was going well so I gently disabused her of that fact. She said Dr Relax had been asking every day. Managed to hold off from crying until the end. Will it ever stop? D-day tomorrow. Well not really as I already know the answer, but final confirmation.

At every failure, especially these big ones it feels like another part of me is dying. Another bit of hope chipped away.

20 November. Pregnancy Test Day. As I now know the terminology – a not very surprising BFN (Big Fat Negative). I don't really feel anything – just numb and tired of it all. Phoned and left a message for Judith and the clinic. This time, the clinic did actually call back and I managed not to cry (quite a result). They offered counselling but I said no, no more.

So, after the failed ICSI, Jason is now in charge. I was really worried that he would just go for the let's get pissed every night, just relax and have lots and lots of sex but he really has thought it through and we are now doing a new set of rules, getting a follow up appointment with Sami David and I am going to see Magda to get herbs and see a healer (that our next door neighbour recommended).   Having said that there are days when I really think a get pissed and forget trying would absolutely be the best way forward; if only I could just forget.

Once again, we are heading in opposite directions, he is now more positive – thinking we have cracked it by having some frozen embryos for once; I am feeling more ground-down than ever and wondering how much more I can take.

But, onward and upward I guess:

Ten things to focus on

1.   Food: good healthy food with lots of vegetables
2.   Drink: less alcohol and more water
3.   Exercise: at least 30 minutes a day and include yoga and qi gong
4.   Western medicine: Sami David's prescriptions and tests and thyroxine
5.   Supplements: Zita West vitamins (vitamin D, folic acid and Omega 3), iron and chlorella
6.   Chinese herbs
7.   Acupuncture

8.   Mental: live with your heart, trust your instincts, leave it to the
      universe

9.   Always have a good book to read

10.   Use music/podcasts to occupy mind

9

Panic

"This, too, shall pass."

Attar of Nishapur

It's fair to say I didn't really take to therapy. Maybe that was just me. Maybe I just didn't find the right therapist. I did find it helpful to have an outlet to talk about all the things swirling round my head which I genuinely felt were starting to drive me clinically insane and to be fair to the various therapists and counsellors, there was no answer (other than the very obvious: get pregnant). I tried all that yoga (apparently stress causes the body to become acidic and yoga breathing helps alkalise the body), Pilates, relaxation shit but I hate going that slowly, it just winds me up not calms me down. I'm also not a big fan of farting in a room full of other people (i.e. yoga class). And I don't think there is anything in the world that would have been able to take my mind off it all and "relax".

But I had started talking to myself (out loud). So, something needed to be done. I muttered sarcastic remarks to myself about pretty much everything (Jason, people taking too long at cash points, the traffic, anyone in my way, and of course, pregnant women, especially belly rubbing pregnant women).

Things then got a bit worse. One day, I had been up, working since 5 am, I was on a short fuse, angry with everyone and everything from the moment I woke up. Thoughts of work, hating work, having too much work to do just swirling round and round my head. So that's the reason nothing is working, all you do is work, work, work. I nipped to Boots to get something. I spotted a woman who had done some reflexology for me. I really, really didn't want to talk to her so I was busy trying to skulk away when she cornered me by the prescriptions counter. I muttered something and just fled, the tears already starting to flow. I don't know why. Judgemental Therapist was right, they were just always so close to the surface.

I thought that was it. At least I had gotten away. But no, she chased me out into the street, bless her, desperate to check if I was okay. I wanted to scream, "No, I'm not fucking okay, but just leave me alone. If I wanted to stay and chat about it, I would have stayed and chatted about it." To add insult to injury, she had her child in tow.

That evening, I mentioned it to Jason, looking for a hug, some empathy. He just intoned, "you'll be fine".

"And what if I'm not?"

"You're strong, you can do it, you'll be fine."

But actually, I really, really don't think I am fine. I really don't think I can keep doing this; keep going. One of the things making me really not fine is how hard I'm finding it to talk to him, how much he doesn't seem to get this, how far apart we seem to be and how tired and lonely that makes me feel. There's the ache of not having children, the ache of not being able to get pregnant, and the ache of having the person you thought you loved and who you thought "got" you, seemingly on a different planet.

10

Healing

"Two roads diverged in a wood, and I, I took the one less travelled by, and that has made all the difference."

Robert Frost

The healer was on Jason's list, so, off I went.

Ok, so the "crazy" stuff/faith/angels etc. isn't really my thing. I went along with the expectation that it would be mostly mumbo jumbo but sod it, I'd tried everything else so why not this as well. And amazingly, he actually made a lot of sense. He didn't ask for any details about my history or even why I was there before we started, instead, I laid down (fully clothed) on a physio bed and he hovered a crystal on a string up and down me. Yes, seriously. After about a minute he asked if there had been something that happened about 4/5 years ago (which would make it 2005/6 – the year we started trying, the year of the start of rows about alcohol, the finding of endometriosis, the beginning of the despair that it wouldn't ever happen).

So 1-0 to the crazy people. Then it was on to what was wrong – and what a list: all my hormones - haywire/shut down; my lymphatic system - shut down; my thyroid gland and thymus - shut down; adrenal and endocrine system - shut down; the bottom chamber of my left lung - mucus; my uterus - not enough progesterone, so not enough endometrium, causing pain as there is nothing for embryos to embed in; the section between the large intestine and the small intestine - blocked; and a section of the intestine wall burnt off from acid; low zinc and folic acid; spinal cord - totally blocked meaning that the hypothalamus can't do its job properly because it can't link down to the coccyx – so the energy is blocked. This was also the cause of the trapped nerve in my left leg; multiple mental issues (we'll get to those later); relatively low blood cells (but generally good blood); bad previous lives which are spilling over into this one; some bad elements in this life.

On the mental side: a small sub-conscious, so mostly a conscious existence – not necessarily a good thing it would appear and a blockage or "blob" between the conscious and sub-conscious – meaning that they don't relate to each other. In terms of emotions: self-pity; guilt; low self-esteem; lack of confidence; desperate to please others; indecision; shame; confusion; aloneness; loneliness; sad; anger; frustration; anxiety; nervous. But apart from that, everything is fine…oh, sorry, I forgot, I also try and force things; I do too much and I don't respect or love myself. Wow.

He did, without prompting, say a number of things which, if I had listened to others, I would have already taken on board. He also said a number of things that were more on the crazy side but still made sense. So, something major (and bad) also happened in 1999 which was the year I started work as a lawyer and realised I had made a terrible career choice; the year I was so worried about money, that despite working at a global law firm I would buy a loaf of bread on Monday morning and see how long I could eek it out to save money but also the year that I met Jason; and when I was 6 or 7 and also before I was born. And the last time I had been truly myself/happy was at 21. He also told me my blood pressure and red and white blood count. Just from a crystal. Oh, and a piece of string.

Despite all of the above, he had, apparently, managed to wipe my slate clean; so it is now for me to take care of me.

I wondered if this was just a hurl and hope approach, mention some medical sounding things, mention some random dates, something has to stick (just like a horoscope). But I was too far gone with this whole thing to care, I decided to just go with it and at least take away from it what I could.

So – things I need to do:

- Love myself
- Believe that I am the most important person and take care of me
- Listen to my intuition
- Lead with my heart (and my head will follow)
- Give in to the universe (hand over baby things to it and then let it do its job – without worrying about it/trying to interfere)
- Do good things (pay it forward)

- Not do too much
- Have fun/do the things I enjoy and not the things I don't
- Don't care what other people think – they are entitled to their opinion
- Wear what I want to wear
- Be who I want to be
- Say no

It was definitely time that I reclaimed that confident happy person I had been. I certainly wasn't perfect – I did worry about things, I was mean sometimes, I said the wrong things or did the wrong things but I always tried to do my best. I had been the person who didn't smoke when everyone else did because they thought it was cool and I thought it was disgusting; I used to wear different colour nail polish on each finger; I had had views on everything from ethics to religion, politics and the economy and I used to believe in voicing them.

So what happened to that person? In part, although I loved university I think the niggling thought (that I wasn't bright enough to be there) became the dominant theme so that even by the time I did pretty well in my finals it was somehow as if it must have been a fluke (hard work; not intelligence); then came work and sadly I took to the competitive nature of a law firm like a duck to water. I can work harder than anyone here; I will do what they want; week one – I will proofread all night because I haven't the guts or common sense to ask when they need it by or push back; I can do everything – be the best.

The cracks were there from day 3 of traineeship (that'll be 1999). Standing looking out over the vast floor of lawyers beavering away and I asked myself why hadn't I had the guts to do anything else. There was no reply. So I pushed on – I must be able to make it work. How long did I have to cry and hate it before I quit – 5 years.

Then I added a barn conversion; the financial drain, a smallholding with over a hundred animals at times, a 4 hour commute and playing sport for my country (granted a pretty minor sport but still) and finally, the pushing to have a baby. And then I pushed for partnership. And again the crying, hating everyday but pushing on – I can do it. And, love him as much as I do (and I do), a relationship in which we take the piss out of each other is great if you have the confidence to take it; but can quickly become very destructive if you don't. It was like having the voice of authority, the person you trust the most, validating all the negative, destructive thoughts in your own head.

But I had been pushing at the wrong things. I do enjoy being busy; I do enjoy working hard, getting things done, doing physical things – but I definitely need to learn when to stop. And to say no.

He may have talked about angels and psychic healing and stuff that would normally make me scoff, wonder about the type of crazy people who believed in all this nonsense but in many ways the healer was spot on. I needed to get back to loving myself, to being myself. Sadly it appeared that that didn't mean treating myself to Belgian buns everyday (which had always been my go-to solution before when I was feeling down) but valuing my opinions, my intellect, my problem solving, my achievements.

11

Pain beyond measure

"Let me not pray to be sheltered from dangers, but to be fearless in facing them. Let me not beg for the stilling of my pain, but for the heart to conquer it."

Rabindranath Tagore

Another of Dr Sami David's recommendations was to have an endometrial biopsy to rule out chronic endometritis (not endometriosis). How bad could it be right? Well, to be honest, whether it was going to hurt or not had not even crossed my mind. An endometrial biopsy was now on the list; it was something that would help and you never know, I might just have it and then that could be the whole reason and I could knock it off the list, take some drugs or do whatever was required to get rid of it and get on with the whole thing.

I spoke to the nice lady in the andrology department (the one who had done the post coital test) who pointed out that they, "deal with all things sperm" (literally, those were her words) and therefore I would need to see someone else to get the elusive biopsy done. She recommended someone at another clinic just round the corner. So off I went.

As always, it started with a consultation, an hour of telling the same story. Amazingly I managed not to cry (wow, I must be getting better at this…). Having assured me that she could do it there and then, weirdly she then suddenly changed her mind and said that first I had to do a pregnancy test which she would have to send off which, of course, meant that I had to come back later.

Not to be deterred we agreed that she would call with the results and then fit me in between her afternoon appointments; apparently it was a quick process so wouldn't take too long.

So back I popped later that day. Usual procedure: lose the bottom half of your clothing, pop up on the bed, attempt to use a small piece of white cloth to cover your dignity, spread your legs and let the nice lady insert some arcane looking device which will be the answer to 5 and half years of agony. She began by saying that it would feel like a smear test to start with and then there would be just a bit of pain and that she needed to get three samples to make sure there was enough so that there would definitely be a result.

Sure enough, in went the device, same slight pain that you get with a smear test. Then it started, searing horrific scraping sucking pain. As if someone was literally tearing my insides out. Tear, suck, tear, suck. My breath started to come quickly and I looked away, biting my lip, hoping it would be over soon. I thought I was good with pain. Thinking that it was at least over, Evil Vampire Doctor (as she shall henceforth be called) calmly, even cheerily, mentioned, "that was the first of the three".

The panic started to rise and my breath came faster. I tried to calm it down, focusing on the wall and hoping that it would soon be over. More tearing and sucking. More ripping from inside out; flesh being sucked off the walls of my insides.

Then it was finally over and Evil Vampire Doctor said I could get dressed and go on my way. I started to put on my skirt but the world narrowed, I was struggling to breathe, I just wanted to get out. I was sweating; profusely. It is running down my face, I reached up and my hair was wet with sweat. If I could just get my clothes on and get out of there but nothing was co-ordinating, my hands were tingling, pins and needles and then throbbing but it was spreading, up my arms and then from my toes and up my legs and I started shaking. And the pain was just ripping through my tummy – waves of it. I wished I could just pass out and it would all stop, at least for a bit.

Evil Vampire Doctor was happily chatting away about something and I knew she had another client waiting (that much had been made patently obvious) so although I wanted out anyway, she clearly also wanted me to go. I sat down on the end of the bed and hoped it would pass quickly so I could finish dressing. Finally, I relinquished and muttered that I wasn't sure I could move just yet. She pulled back the curtain and told me to lie down. She then left and I tried to reach my phone to call Jason. I didn't get through and for the first time ever, in all my hospital visits (and there had been a lot) I was truly scared. It felt like things were shutting down and I just wanted to speak to him, to tell him that I love him and apologise for pushing for all this.

A nurse came in before I could try and get dressed again and started muttering about everything being just fine. Maybe a cup of tea would help. I let one leg slip off the bed, trying to find something cold.

They decided I needed to move, there was after all the other patient who needed the bed. Still only half-dressed they gave me another piece of small white cloth to wrap around me while I went down the corridor to another room. The cloth didn't even meet at the back but I didn't care anymore. The room turned out to be their mini surgery room so had one of those beds with the top half upright so you can't actually lie down on it. I therefore lay, half on, half off the bed, with legs dangling off the end of it. The nurse mentioned that it didn't look very comfortable but she didn't know how to put the other part down. Brilliant. She went off in search of a biscuit. Ten minutes later she was back with two wrapped chocolates. She offered me one but I was still shaking so much it took a while to open it. When I finally managed it, it did taste good and I think the sugar helped. In the meantime, she had tucked into the other one (I didn't realise we were having a tea party together) and reportedly enjoyed it (so that was a relief). She then said that this happens all the time and I really shouldn't worry about it.

Worry about it? It felt like the fucking world was ending, literally. If this happens all the time then there is something seriously wrong. How can they be licensed to carry out these kinds of procedures with not a sedative in sight, let alone an anaesthetic; with only a mention of "brief" pain?

After about 20 minutes the shaking had stopped and sweat receded and I really just needed to get out of there. After 4 more attempts I managed to leave a message for Jason – yes, he was in a meeting and not picking up but the female voice for his voicemail message was at least familiar. I started crying. The nurse went out for something and I got dressed. Well I started to get dressed and then realised that when they brought my things through they had forgotten to bring my skirt. The nurse came back, with the skirt, thankfully. Dressed, I finally left. The pain had almost totally stopped, the sweating had stopped and I wandered down the road, £670 lighter, wondering what the hell had just happened.

12

Control

"It's like in the great stories, Mr. Frodo. The ones that really mattered. Full of darkness and danger they were. And sometimes you didn't want to know the end…because how could the end be happy? How could the world go back to the way it was when so much bad had happened? But in the end, it's only a passing thing…this shadow. Even darkness must pass."

J.R.R. Tolkien, Lord of the Rings

The frustration at the lack of control was just immense.

As an illustration, my GP is lovely (most of the time) and had been very helpful. I went to her and asked for Clomid. I already had had some from Dr Helpful but Critical but it had expired and as one last desperate attempt as money was getting tight I thought why not – a little boost would do no harm. So I asked for a prescription. And then I got the impression that was really not the done thing. But, fair play, she said she would ask Doctor Relax. Which, in the age of the internet, clearly demanded that a letter be written and a response be waited for. Seven weeks later she called me in for a review. And handed me the written response. Which was dated 4 weeks previously. It very kindly noted how sorry he was that I was still not pregnant. He went on in his own inimical way to state that, "particularly with unexplained subfertility continuing to try to conceive spontaneously is not necessarily fruitless although the longer the period of subfertility exists then the less likely it is that this will occur. It is appropriate therefore to try to find a balance between giving some cause for hope and at the same time not necessarily giving unrealistic expectations." And it then lamented that as there was no empirical evidence requiring the use of Clomid; no such prescription could be given as, fuck me, it could result in a multiple pregnancy.

I wanted to scream: Yes, I have read of the statistics which will tell you that a multiple birth is more dangerous. I am fully aware of those studies. I am also fully aware that part of the IVF process is about playing the odds and that they, almost invariably, put back two embryos. They also stuff you full of drugs, the long-term side effects of which are arguably still unknown; they readily put you under general anaesthetic; and they let you wallow in a pit of despair, self-loathing; depression and suicidal desires; but one prescription that promotes ovulation. No, no, no, no, no. Certainly not for you, Mrs. Infertile. We need empirical evidence first. I tell you what; go away; actually do some research on this entire area (and not just research on how to make the IVF process more streamlined so you can charge more and process patients faster but some actual research on why so many women can't get pregnant naturally) and then come back and tell me I can't have one lousy fucking prescription for Clomid. I really didn't mean to take it out on my GP but Dr Relax was not in the room and to my shame I found it impossible to hide my disgust and anger.

By now there had been 70 periods and no pregnancy. Not even close. I was starting to feel like I had reached rock bottom.

I had spent six years of what should have been the prime of my life, deeply depressed, very, very angry, bitter, resentful and suicidal. That's not quite fair - there had been days and times at which, and I never thought I would say this, but that I was grateful. Grateful that all of this had pulled me up short and made me realise what I did have; that I couldn't always have what I wanted and I needed to accept that; that I couldn't control everything. Grateful that it had made be reassess who I was and where I was going. I would never, in a million years have thought I would be someone who self-harmed and I hadn't, but I had come pretty close. I'd felt utter revulsion at myself; a deep desire to cut out those parts of me that didn't or wouldn't work. I'd felt an urge, a reflex which demanded I cause physical pain to match the mental, to punish myself for failing. I didn't know if what I'd felt was depression but it certainly felt fucking awful and inescapable – no matter how much I battled in my head and fought to bring myself back to rationality; there was such an inevitability to the dark thoughts.

I don't know why there but it was always at Embankment Tube, waiting for the District or Circle line. For about 18 months, every working day, I would stand near the edge (in front of the yellow line – the part where all the pushy, "busy and important" people stand because getting on the Tube is more important than their own safety). It was always there. I would stand and look down and contemplate the small step it would take to be rid of the pain, to stop the constant voice in my head, to shut it off. I'm not sure if I really wanted to die but I did so, so desperately want the pain to end.

13

Hope

"If you're going through hell, keep going."

Winston Churchill

"Getting over a painful experience is much like crossing the monkey bars. You have to let go at some point in order to move forward."

C.S. Lewis

The crying was relentless and just utterly exhausting. I don't think I actually cried every day but it was damn close. If you add up crying multiple times in one day then I guess it was pretty much every day for six years. At times it really helped to cry but it was exhausting and in itself made me angry. Why could I not just deal with this situation?

I cried when I found out a friend was pregnant (usually at home, on my own). I cried when friends gave birth. I cried, a lot, every time the IVF failed. I cried every time I got my period. I cried every time I felt the utter hopelessness of the situation crushing down on me.

It had been creeping up on me for a long time. If I am honest part of it was also because with Jason in charge I was no longer thinking about what step was next – the only steps which were next were the next month, the next month of trying to have sex at the right time, feeling pressure to have sex all the time, oh and of course relaxing (that after all being the only thing I needed to get right) and then waiting for my period to come. Which it always did. So, what was the fucking point? I no longer even felt like I might get pregnant. I no longer felt there was hope that this month might be the month. I just wanted to drink to oblivion.

It may also have been the discussions we had started having about surrogacy (by 2011 I got in touch with clinics in the US, Thailand and India about the process and costs). Proper discussions, not just the silly, what a relief no stretch marks, pain of childbirth, morning sickness discussions. In part, I didn't really care if that was the way we went, other than the fact that it obviously costs a lot of money; it would give us children.

I was at the point where I didn't even want to kill myself or harm myself anymore. Incredibly, that now seemed like too much effort. I was so, so desperately tired of it all.

I had thought I could and would fight everything to the end, but now I just felt defeated. It was like I was in the last five minutes of a game, I was still chasing and harrying but the difference in the score line was just too great and I had that feeling in the pit of my stomach that it didn't matter how hard I fought; it was over. The clock was running down but now I was just going through the motions, somehow playing for pride.

I think I was starting to, not accept in the true sense, but believe that I was just someone who couldn't or would just never have kids. I signed up with the Tony Robbins coaching programme – partly a desperate attempt to try and live a more controlled life. Most of what they do is centered on having a big vision for your life and then making it happen. I would always have said children were that vision but now they are so distant it seemed crazy even to include them – it was like saying my vision is to win the lottery when I don't even play.

14

The Lists

"Listen to the MUSTN'TS, child

Listen to the DON'TS

Listen to the SHOULDN'TS, the IMPOSSIBLES, the WON'TS

Listen to the NEVER HAVES, then listen close to me -

Anything can happen, child.

ANYTHING can be."

Shel Silverstein

After trying for so long, I had accumulated lists of all things to do and not do in order to get pregnant. No, correction, they were the lists of things to do and not do to **try** (very important that distinction) and get pregnant. Every day. I had this crazy theory that if I didn't do one of them well enough or if I did do one of those things that I wasn't supposed to, then it would all go wrong and I would also have to deal with the guilt and worry that I had screwed it all up and then the guilt and worry about feeling guilty and worrying, aaaargh…

1. Relax – at all times, judging from the amount of times people told me this (from paid professionals to those who were offering friendly advice) I'm guessing it is the number one priority

2. Have sex – at the right times, in the right positions

3. Have sex everyday from day 16

4. Take your temperature every morning, before you move (apart from to pick the thermometer up off the floor. Note to self, don't drop it)

5. Pee on a stick, every morning to see whether the fertility monitor thinks you are even vaguely ovulating or not

6. Eat red meat (but also see point 30 below, and 23)

7. Have acupuncture

8. Repeat the mantra: I am healthy and fertile, and my hormones are balanced

9. Have cranial osteopathy

10. Use Chinese herbs

11. Exercise (but not too much or too long; not enough to get an endorphin high)

12. Stay positive (at all times)

13. Believe in the power of the universe

14. Keep your feet warm at all times

15. Keep your belly warm at and post ovulation

16. Get between 7 and 8 hours sleep every night

17. Drink at least 10 glasses of water a day

18. Drink room temperature filtered water; not tap water and not water that is too cold

19.   Eat lots and lots of vegetables

20.   Pan pipes (courtesy of Jason's mother) – apparently forget everything else, just play pan pipes. I wasn't sure if it was supposed to be during sex or just generally but I decided it was best not to ask.

21.   Believe each month that you will get pregnant (despite all evidence to the contrary)

22.   Enjoy sex, at all times, even if it is the last thing you want to do

23.   Do things that contradict other things e.g. it is late, in order to get at least 7 hours sleep you need to go to sleep now but you also need to have sex, which needs to be slow enough that you can have it without it hurting but quick enough to still tick the sleep box

24.   Be enormously pleased for everyone that is either pregnant or has just had a baby

25.   Sympathise endlessly with anyone who has morning sickness or sleepless nights

26.   Take false unicorn root (that's when you know you have really lost the plot)

27.   Eat more fibre, especially in week 4 (implantation time)

28.   Chew your food lots

29.   Eat before 8.30 pm

30.   Only eat meat three times a week

31.   Eat 6 to 7 portions of vegetables a day

The Do Nots

1.   Use tin foil

2.   Use cling film

3. Hold a mobile phone within 6 feet (or was it meters?) of yourself at all times (not sure how you are supposed to make calls but maybe now is the time to go back to the landline only)

4. Eat red meat (yes, it is also on the Do List, see no. 23 of the Do List)

5. Drink alcohol

6. Stay up late

7. Drink any caffeinated drinks

8. Eat sugar

9. Touch cat pee (this one really is true)

10. Eat processed food

11. Use chemical cleaning products

12. Feel stressed about anything at any time (although subsequent research has shown stress to be just what is needed, see no. 23 of the Do List)

13. Use deodorant with aluminium (i.e. don't use deodorant other than random rock crystal shit which doesn't stop you sweating or smelling despite having the pleasure of enabling you to spend three times as much as you would on normal deodorant)

14. Use tampons – use a moon cup. OMG.

15. Have oral sex

16. Use a microwave, I've never worked out if this meant that you shouldn't eat microwaved food or just not stand in front of a microwave, or was it both?

17. Take painkillers. I think paracetamol might be okay but probably best not, just to be on the safe side.

18. Eat white food

1. Quinoa
2. Brown rice
3. Apple cider vinegar
4. Miso soup
5. Tempeh (I have no idea what that even is)
6. Tamari (ditto)
7. Mushrooms
8. Sesame, pumpkin, sunflower seeds
9. Green tea
10. Fennel
11. Rosemary
12. Parsnips
13. Onions
14. Leeks
15. Artichokes
16. Thyme, basil, garlic, mint
17. Apricots
18. Chicken
19. Goat's yoghurt and cheese
20. Linseed
21. Alkaline foods
22. Wheatgrass tablets or powder (is that not processed?)
23. Sea greens (seriously?)
24. Fish oil
25. Flaxseed oil

26.   Hemp seeds

27.   Turkey

28.   Apples (also see below)

29.   Beetroot

30.   Pears

31.   Peppers

32.   Grapes

33.   Citrus fruit

34.   Squash

35.   Garlic

36.   Beans/pulses

The food not to eat/eat less of/things not to drink or drink less of

1.   Anything with preservatives/chemicals

2.   Fried food

3.   Fatty food

4.   Acidic foods (and the apple cider vinegar?)

5.   Diary (where does that leave the goat's yoghurt and cheese?)

6.   Flax seeds/linseed (but see nos. 20 and 25 in the list above)

7.   Alcohol

8.   Fruit juice

9.   Refined sugar

10.   Raw food/cold food/frozen food (especially in ovulation phase)

11.   Tofu/processed soya

12.   Couscous

13.   Apples (er…)

14.   Broccoli

15. Spinach

16. Peaches

17. Pears (also er...)

18. Turnips

19. Peanuts

Exercise

1. Phase 1 (menstruation I've always hated that word even before all this): low impact if your period is heavy. Otherwise, aerobic but not too intense. Include a meditative component.

2. Phase 2: no idea

3. Phase 3 (ovulation): daily gentle exercise

4. Phase 4 (implantation): moderate aerobic, keep your energy high

Other required steps

1. A hot water bottle, 20 minutes per evening, in first half of cycle.

2. 20 minutes of sunlight a day (to activate the pituitary gland function)

3. Don't eat too late (there should be 3-4 hours between eating and going to bed – so supper on the train on the way home from work then?)

4. Relaxation techniques (especially around ovulation and possible implantation)

5. Meditation, deep breathing

6. Laugh and have fun (obligatory)

7. Avoid frustrations (what, like inability to get pregnant?)

8. Do one thing a day for you

9. Self massage

10. Visualisation

11. Don't overdo work (but still find money to pay for crazy treatments)

12. Rest

13. Regular bedtime

14. Wear bed socks

15. Write down your goals (easy – GET PREGNANT)

16. Say no

17. Set limits with people

18. Protect your back by bending your knees (all the time?)

Testing

And lists of tests to have before you spend even more money on procedures:

APA (antiphospholipid antibodies)

Prolactin

Karyotypes (chromosome)

Post coital

Immunobead binding blood test

Thrombophilia

Serial progesterone

PCOS

Genito-urinary

And lists of some of the pills and potions I thought I should take at any one time and some I foisted on Jason:

Me:

Vitamin D3

Primrose Oil

Mucus Cough Menthol

Zinc

Lecithin

Chromium Picolinate

Vitex agnus – castus

Royal Jelly

Wheatgrass

Chromium

L'arginine

Carnitine

Glutamine powder

Echinacea tincture

Aloe Vera juice

Liquid Algae

Smokeless Moxa (it may say it is smokeless but in fact it wasn't and I also managed to burn a hole in the sheets and bedroom floor with it – so best to have a fire extinguisher at the ready)

Pregnacare Plus Omega 3

Pregnacare Conception

Cranberry juice

Folic Acid

Vitamin E

Chlorella

Co-enzyme Q10

Selenium

Nickel

Vitamin B complex

Magnesium

Calcium

EPO – omega 6

Red raspberry leaf (in fact I rarely took this as I was so scared it would be a problem if, God forbid, I did ever get pregnant)

Low dose aspirin

Calcichew D3 Forte

Milk Thistle

Spirula

Jason:

ASC Plus (no longer available in the UK but thank you internet)

Wellman conception

Selenium plus zinc

As the herbalist had noted, it was insane to be taking such a vast array of vitamins and potions but that was part of the problem – I had lost all perspective, and in my desperation to find something that worked, I ended up trying everything. So, I certainly wouldn't in any way advise anyone to follow these lists; in fact if anything I'd suggest the opposite – don't do what I did and instead simplify where possible and don't get caught up in the minutiae.

Jason and I discussed the various ways in which clinics fuck things up. No. Stop. New leaf. Trying to swear less and be more positive: what I meant to say was ways in which they could do things better:

1. Do **NOT** put the fertility unit next to the pregnancy/maternity ward.

2. In fact, supermarkets – please, please do not put the tampons and those disgusting things called sanitary pads next to the pregnancy tests and fertility "aids" or the fucking baby aisle. It is bad enough having to admit to yourself that your period means another month of failure without having to wade through a bunch of new mothers with that smug proud way they have and fucking babies and pictures of babies everywhere. Would you put the condoms and lynx next to the impotence drugs – no, so don't do the female equivalent.

3. But back to IVF clinics – do <u>NOT</u> allow people with children to wait in the same area – in fact if you possibly can, ban people from bringing their small children when attending the hospital/clinic and if you do have a sign asking them to wait in another waiting room actually fucking enforce it.

4. Warn patients that they will need to buy sanitary pads during the two week wait – just in case – unless you have some deal going on with DFS/John Lewis with a discount on new bed linen and mattresses.

5. If you don't get the pain that a patient feels and let's face it, unless you've been through it you don't (which is completely understandable), then acknowledge you can't imagine how they feel or at least don't keep telling them not to worry about it.

6.   Ask if they want information and if the answer is yes – give them everything – as much detail as you possibly can.

7.   Structure scans and blood tests so they actually follow each other without a 45-minute (aka 2 hour) gap between the two.

8.   If you need more than one waiting room (other than for those people with children with them) you have a problem with scheduling and/or staffing.

9.   The waiting rooms – they just suck – they should provide privacy not the opposite. If you call out names use first names – some people haven't told their closest friends or family and yet their full names ring out loud and clear to rooms full of other people. Often the reception desk is nearby or the nurses are so loud and indiscrete that the world and his wife knows Jill Smith is about to have a scan/transfer/blood test and John Smith is about to pop along to that room down the corridor and wank into a pot, not too fast, not too slow, over some very old and bad porn mags.

10.   Porn – variety – there are more porn magazines out there than Escort (apparently). Get a regular supply of different titles.

11.   Stop taking the piss out of blokes who are scared shitless of blood tests. Yes, they are absolute wusses and in the grand scheme of all that a woman goes through, they seriously need to suck it up and get on with it but at the same time, it is a physical and very visceral fear – so pander to them. They will be eternally grateful.

12.   If you do have a lot of people to see maybe, I don't know, open for more hours a day or even at the weekend (yes, both days) so you don't have people sitting, waiting, for hours. It might also make it

feel less like a production line. It might mean your staff actually recognise people they have asked to remove half their clothes and taken blood from three times in a week.

13. Ditch the baby pictures, every last fucking one of them. PLEASE. They don't help. They just taunt and goad.

14. Do transfers and egg collections on days which fit the patient's medical needs, not your staffing schedule.

15. Have more than one receptionist or a telephone overflow system that means patients speak to a person not a voicemail message. Respond to voicemails and missed calls. If you are calling from work, you get seconds before someone disturbs you/you have to get back to your desk – the stress of having to find another free moment really doesn't help. Or – use email (revolutionary….).

16. Be honest about the chances of success, but at the same time you don't have to ram the chance of failure down people's throats.

17. Do **<u>NOT</u>** mention the word "luck" – do not, repeat, not, tell someone who has handed you responsibility for their life's dreams and hopes (as well as roughly £6k a go), that they were unlucky – it isn't correct and it really, really doesn't help. Talk statistics, talk science, talk reassurance about a course of treatment but do not label someone as unlucky.

18. Accept credit cards.

19. Do not inflate the drug charges. Or make people buy more drugs than they need.

15

Sperm

"When you get into a tight place and everything goes against you, till it seems as though you could not hold on a minute longer, never give up then, for that is just the place and time that the tide will turn."

Harriet Beecher Stowe

A chance conversation with a former boss led him to tell me that his sister and her husband had been to Israel for treatment for her husband who produced no sperm at all. He insisted I call her. I ignored him.

Jason produced more sperm than a whale and had been repeatedly told by allegedly top men in their field, that his sperm was perfect. In fact, Dr Perfect had gone even further, "maybe don't get plastered every night of the week (said in that bromance, wink, wink, nudge, nudge, we all enjoy a pint down the pub, we men who know how to take our drink) but apart from that drink as much as you wish because it will make no difference."

Now I had always thought it slightly odd that having an undescended testicle as a child which required a corrective operation did not seem to be considered relevant to sperm producing equipment but then I'm a girl and a very emotional one who knows fuck all about these matters so who am I to ask difficult questions? Plus, not a single doctor (other than Dr David) had ever asked anything about testicles during all our appointments so they must be irrelevant. Right?

Fast forward five years. There had been that sperm test which resulted in ICSI being required. Things were no longer looking entirely perfect. And besides, the longer it went on the more I looked and looked for anything that might just be the key or even the 1% change that made all the difference.

I called my boss' sister.

And she told me about varicoceles. It is a bit like having varicose veins in your testicles (as I understand it) and apparently it occurs in around 15% of men. And it is often discovered when investigating male infertility. Boss' sister's husband had it and he had it fixed and hey presto, pregnancy shortly followed.

I mentioned the "miracle" cure from Israel to Jason, not expecting much response. Instead he offered to go for the scan – well ok, maybe not offered but he didn't fight it tooth and nail which in my book equates to the same thing. Off he went for the scan. I had been led to believe, genuinely, that the scan was just that – lie there, put up with the noise, get big equipmenty thing to take pictures, come home. Well it turned out that

116

in fact there was actually a fair amount of feeling up of his balls, and not in a good way. Fuck me, compared to having the inside of your cervix cauterised, repeatedly scraped and then slices taken out of it I think a little ball feeling should be acceptable but maybe that is just me.

We weren't expecting anything but when the results come through later that day, there was varicoceles in both testicles. It was noted like it was an everyday occurrence. It probably is if you spend your entire working life feeling up balls.

At this stage we had been trying for just over 6 years. To be absolutely correct, 72 months. 72 periods. 3 operations. 2 rounds of IVF. 1 round of ICSI. Approximately £20k in private health care costs. Numerous consultations with "top" doctors on Harley Street. And a "top" doctor in the US. I had been advised (and had) changed my job; my entire lifestyle. I had tried homeopathy; reflexology; acupuncture; Chinese herbs; moxi sticks; nutritionists (x 2); cranial osteopathy; massage; counselling. I had had suicidal feelings for over 18 months; rows with Jason so violent my throat hurt from shouting; we had drowned ourselves in alcohol; we had lived "clean"; no sugar; no diary; no alcohol; no processed foods; we had tried sex every day; sex every other day; sex every three days; sex up to a point and then no sex; sex at different times of the day; sex and then lying still; sex and then lying still with bottom raised. I had done exercise; no exercise; yoga; qui gong; running; not more than gentle jogging. I had had room temperature water only; vitamins; cut the hair off the back of my head for hair analysis tests; more internal and external investigations than you could shake a stick at; been poked and prodded in all directions. I had taken my temperature every morning; peed on sticks every morning; saved piss in a cup if I was in a different time zone; held "funerals" in my head after every failed IVF because I was told that would help and there is no body to bury; I had, at least in public, been happy for every other fucking person who had a baby; I had tried being more feminine; wearing make-up; dressing more femininely; felt for my own cervix opening; assessed whether it was an end of nose tip or a chin dimple; taken drugs galore; vitamins; cough medicine; taken Clomid and not taken Clomid when it had been refused due to lack of empirical evidence. But aside from the sperm tests and some questions from Dr David there had not been a single fucking question about my husband's sperm, lifestyle or medical history. Not one. Ever. And definitely no questions about his actual testicles.

It seemed the only doctor in the world who had pioneered a procedure to address it in a non-invasive way was based in Israel and the procedure costs $13.5k and when asked of chances of success (which I did by email) his extraordinary response was "God willing". Seriously…

Then, from a chance enquiry, luck did seem to be on our side. As it turned out there was a doctor not a million miles away, in fact, about 12 miles away, who was completely willing and able to do a varicocele embolization (as I now knew it was called), on the NHS. WTF.

16

Things not to do if I ever get pregnant/have a baby

Or

Top tips for those with friends who can't get pregnant/have a baby – please, please don't….

"Don't wait. The time will never be just right."

Napoleon Hill

Okay, I just like lists – so here are a few more…

DON'T:

1. Wear the world's tightest tops, stretched so tight that someone at 100m could tell if my belly button is an inny or outy.

2.	Buy a yellow plastic sign for the car with a grating, smug note about there being a baby, little princess, bump, special twat on board. Just likely to result in infertile women wanting to ram my car more.

3.	Smile smugly at single or childless women staring at me.

4.	Rub belly, repeatedly especially when aforesaid women are staring.

5.	Look around expectantly on the underground, rubbing belly/arching back.

6.	Send photos of newly born child to anyone other than people who ask/parents. This applies whether covered in mucus, bodily fluids or clean.

7.	Ditto pictures of scans (at whatever stage).

8.	Ditto details of mucus plug giving way/waters breaking. Seriously, what is wrong with these people…

9.	Breast-feed, repeatedly or indeed at all, in front of people without children.

10.	Talk, mention, even mutter about how hard pregnancy is.

11.	Ditto the difficulties of having small children.

12.	Ditto sleepless nights.

13.	Ditto about costs of buying new things for the precious one.

14.	Tell anyone to relax about getting pregnant, or indicate that that is, after all, all they need to do.

15.	Tell anyone it will just happen – if they just have faith.

My baby commandments

1.	Never give up

2.	There is always hope

3.	Be strong

1. Everything is relative
2. Every cloud has a silver lining: it's not a horrific period day and the end of all hope – it is day 1, a new cycle and a new chance. I only ever managed that one when I had had a stiff drink.
3. Do what you feel is right
4. Say no when you should
5. Value yourself, your time, your health
6. Find a distraction: you can't just forget about it but if you can find something, anything, that takes your mind off it all that would help – a rubbish film, a good book
7. Laugh: find something, anything, that makes you laugh

Secrets for life

1. It's okay to ask for and accept help
2. It's okay to accept compliments
3. Give compliments
4. You can control anything by the right mental approach – you can always control your reaction
5. Take the road less travelled

Resolutions

1. Get 7-8 hours sleep a night
2. Be asleep before midnight
3. Drastically reduce sugar
4. Only drink red wine and only one glass with supper

5.   Exercise for one hour 6 days a week

6.   Take vitamins every day

7.   Drink at least 3 litres of water a day

8.   Do pelvic floor exercises 5 times a day

9.   Do yoga once a week (on your own so no one else can hear or smell your farts)

10.   Tidy the house every week while listening to online lectures/talks

11.   Eat vegetarian meals 5 times a week

12.   Eat eggs every day (I hate eggs)

13.   Spend within budget

14.   Complete diary tasks

15.   Fight clean

16.   Act on intuition/instinct

17   Know your own opinion and voice it

18.   Embrace mistakes/failure

19.   Work smart not hard

20.   No guilt

21.   No worrying

22.   Take life less seriously

23.   Sing and dance

17

Rolling the Dice … again

"If you can't fly then run, if you can't run then walk, if you can't walk then crawl, but whatever you do you have to keep moving forward."

Martin Luther King Jr.

Jason's trying naturally programme had still not worked so it was back to IVF. This time we chose the clinic partly on the advice of Gabrielle (if they can make her think they are half decent then they must be amazing) and also on advice of a former acupuncturist – I'm guessing it's not a great sign to be told even by your acupuncturist that there isn't really much more they can do for you. Magda let it slip one day, just when I thought things were actually going well, that "if" I get pregnant – it was just in passing amidst one of her rants about something else but there it was – no more when, no more of course you will (which had always been her style), just IF….

The clinic was also not in London so was cheaper. Off we went. Dr Calm seemed ok. Usual talk about dice. Rolling. Statistics. Blah blah blah. He did say surrogacy was a waste of money, "nothing wrong with your womb, just your chromosomes". So it turns out we can just keep giving them money for repeated IVF attempts – the sky is the limit!

He did express some surprise at Dr Relax's parting words that three attempts were as good as it would get but then, we were sitting there with cheque book in hand. In fact, it was far, far better than that, we were sitting there with a visa card. Woohoo. We could now throw the dice on credit.

Had the two hour "here is how you stick needles in yourself" appointment and to be fair they did seem pretty nice, caring people. Have got the drugs so all systems go on Friday.

I guess the part I still didn't get, although I managed to have a row with Jason about it who clearly thought I was an idiot for not getting it – how can it be that with 3 rounds of IVF and 6 years of trying and a shed load of sex, how can it be that I have never, ever been pregnant – how can there have been a chromosomal defect every time? Are we just that unlucky? Really?

Also, just to add to the fun, I had found a lump or rather a few in my right breast. Not sure if it was just because I had lost weight or something else (over a stone since the lovely Jason told me, "I had let myself go" or rather, "I told you not to let yourself go and look what you've done").

So, off to hospital for tests, several people touching them up, followed by a mammogram, followed by an ultrasound, followed by more touching, followed by we're not sure, probably nothing, please come back for some more in 6 weeks.

I was sure it is nothing. But being in a breast clinic was a rather sobering experience and also just a very stark reminder that I was just trying to get pregnant – I wasn't ill (I hoped) or looking death in the face – I just couldn't have a child. Yet.

17 February. I start Buserlin today, so the rollercoaster starts all over again. It was a bad day for various reasons I won't bore you with but overall, after six years of what I am now admitting to myself is probably some kind of mental health issue, I actually feel better, a lot better. I still wasn't really not looking forward to the cycle not working and the pain and anger but I knew I would survive.

All fine with the injections but it is weird though how some points to inject really hurt and others I can barely feel. I guess it is just distribution of pain receptors.

23 February. After such a promising start, towards the end of the week the bad mood is really starting to kick in and the anger and resentment are back. The thing making it all so much worse is that I really thought I was done with that stage so am bitterly disappointed with myself that I am back in black mood territory.

5 March. Baseline scan: all fine except I am diagnosed with PCOS. Apparently only mild and not a problem. Er....6.5 years of trying and it is the first I have heard of it. WTF (again).

19 March. My skin has gone funny, my tummy looks like a pin cushion and the skin doesn't want to give way – which sounds odd but it is as if the needle isn't sharp enough so as I push the skin just seems to fold in but not yield as if it has put up the defence shield.

Today should have been egg collection day but instead it was another scan. Which was ok. At least things were growing (touch wood). There were 13 follicles on Friday so it looked like Wednesday for collection and Friday or Monday for transfer. There have definitely been some vile moods and a fair dollop of self-pity but actually probably the best cycle in terms of not building up too much hope and just going with it.

But, as ever, I spend a decent amount of time in the waiting rooms. The endless pictures of babies on the walls are deeply, deeply annoying. Would they put pictures of L'Oréal adverts for shampoo on the walls of cancer units – no – so what the fuck are all the baby pictures about – here – while you spend quite literally hours waiting, staring in the face of all that you can't have, all you have failed to achieve. Not enough that you have to do it in your own time – just walking down the street or at weekends with friends; no, come to the one place that can allegedly help and we'll rub it in a bit more. They are literally everywhere, huge collages, on every wall – just when you thought that's it, you turn a corner and there are some more. I guess they think it shows how good they are – stick with us, show us your money and this is our gift to you. I get that but would far rather they showed you that in stats. Not the pictures, not the cute babies staring at you everywhere you turn.

Looking around the waiting room I wonder what hell every other woman has been through. Some look ok; others are very, very busy professional types who clearly don't have time to be waiting (me until very recently); others, just look quite old and worn down. There is quite an air of unspoken sadness.

23 March. Slightly later than expected, I had the egg collection on Wednesday – one slight problem was that they appear to have over-stimulated me so I ended up with 27 follicles. 20 of those released eggs and of those, so far 13 have survived. Jason's sperm must be on the up as they said no need for ICSI, so we saved £1,300 just like that.

However, they are now waiting to see what grows well and what doesn't but with 13 there is a fair chance of some to put back and even possibly some to freeze. So far one is 6 cells – apparently that is bad by this stage so they have discounted that one – weird that speed in these circumstances is a sign of failure but then again maybe I really shouldn't be surprised. Apparently, there is one very good 4 cell, 3 x 3 cell and the rest are 2 cells – so transfer will be Saturday or Monday.

26 March. Transfer day – they told us there was a blastocyst and a morula and they were putting those back in. On the bed. Legs akimbo. Up goes the bed so that my vagina is at the doctor's eye level. Me desperately wishing I had taken Jason's advice and shaved or waxed or something – particularly when he caught one of the hairs on the way in. Ho hum. Do you hold hands at this point? Should I stare at him longingly (Jason that is, not the embryologist – whose eyes I could just see above my paper sarong)? I'm entirely sure so I just stare at the roof tiles and wonder about the clinic's cleaning schedule. In they go and he (embryologist still) tells me to say a little prayer – so instead of relaxing and visualising I then start having an existential debate about whether, as a confirmed atheist I should pray or whether that is really rather rude at this point – you can't just turn God on and off when you wish – that just wouldn't be right. But then again, considering how important this is am I not better to hedge my bets?

All day I could feel things, at least I thought I could. I actually felt pregnant. This could really be it. I could actually be having a child or children. Really finally having children. Then, I'm not sure entirely how it happened – maybe it was my fear that the "feelings of something different" were actually just hunger pangs.   Maybe it was just the hormonal emotional rollercoaster that is the dreaded 2 week wait. Maybe it was lying awake for two hours wondering why my stomach no longer felt hot (just cold, which I now know, because as one acupuncturist kindly pointed out, is due to belly fat). Maybe it was my all-encompassing pessimism rearing its ugly head again. I don't know but that "pregnant feeling" seemed to slip away. By morning it was all but gone.

27 March. They say that implantation will take place 24-72 hours after the transfer. Does that mean that nothing happens in the first 24 hours? Apparently some people have implantation bleeding – according to the internet it is about a third. Implantation bleeding doesn't mean that you are pregnant and you can be pregnant without it.

Then the clinic called – none of the remaining 8 were worth freezing. Forget not top of their maths class or a little slow at learning to speak. My embryos (and apparently they aren't even embryos until they implant, so my blastocyst (which one was), morulas and cells, none of them were even worth giving a chance to; none were worth £600 – the cost of freezing. Maybe that is the price of life - £600. A burger plus fries anyone?

So, from 27 follicles, 20 eggs, 13 fertilised, 8 were very good at day 3 but by day 5 they were all dud bar 2. No wonder we were getting nowhere naturally. I still struggle to understand how anyone gets pregnant naturally and how people seem to do it with such ease.

I guess I was just hoping to increase our insurance policy with some frozen ones and yet, despite being overstimulated that wasn't going to happen. I am kicking myself and telling myself repeatedly that I am incredibly lucky – lots of people don't make it this far; we've never had a blastocyst before; at least we did go to day 5 so we knew which would be the best; at least we can afford to be doing this; thank you credit cards. I keep trying to mentally slap myself and question why I have given myself lower odds (10:90) than even the official statistics. As if by some miracle of reverse psychology I'd be proved wrong in a blaze of wonderful, beautiful babies.

I keep trying to tell myself, "it's not so bad – if it fails, we just go again". And keep going.

I think the thing I just still find hard is not being able to control my own mind. I thought I controlled everything. My mind. My body. My reactions. But apparently not. When will I learn to accept that and just go with it? When will I learn to give in?

28 March. Another day and although still not feeling pregnant I do feel better. Maybe it is just that today the sun is shining and I've come round to the fact that if this one doesn't work we just move to the next round. Maybe it's also because the internet reassured me that straining to poo won't make the embryos pop out. So relief all round.

6 April. Pregnancy test day. Up, peed on the stick. Nothing. I started my by now usual rant about it all being a fucking waste of time and stormed off to get dressed.

Jason called out. What the fuck does he want now? I'm not interested in another consolation hug.

"Look."

"Look at what?"

"The stick."

Me peering at it with the anger rising …. "and?"

"It's positive."

"No it fucking isn't, stop fucking about".

"Is it?"

"There's a faint line. You have to wait for three whole minutes you know," he said in that taking the piss, laughing at me way, which just made me more angry.

"Bollocks."

"There really is a line."

"Show me that thing." Is it? Is it? Could it be? I don't believe it. It was actually quite a strong blue line by now.

"Sainsburys. Now." The only place I could think of that would be open early enough. I bought two more tests.

They all seemed to be positive. I had started trying to get pregnant when I was 30. I was now nearly 37. I sat on the loo and stared into the middle distance in sheer disbelief. And then back at the last stick. Really? The day I never thought would come. Relief and fear flooded my body. What if it is a false positive, what if I miscarry? Oh, just shut up and let yourself just enjoy this moment, right now (according to three tests) you are pregnant. That may change the next time you go to the loo. But right now, in this instant, you are pregnant.

Started crying – it just feels so weird. Rushed to the clinic to get more cyclogest. The nurse was so excited – she said we just looked shell-shocked. We were. Drove over to my mum and dad's who I think were equally shell-shocked. Our hot chocolate thing had become a full blow superstition by now (not sure why when it clearly hadn't worked for cycle

131

no.3) but nevertheless, every appointment we had to stop for a hot chocolate so we carried on; just in case.

7 April. Small amounts of brown spotting. Trying to ignore it.

8 April. More brown spotting. Still trying to think it is nothing.

9 April. I rang the clinic who said if it was brown then nothing to worry about – just your body getting used to the fact that it is pregnant and as long as it doesn't go red then all ok. Just take it easy. No need to stay in bed. Three hours later it was red and there was more. Can't decide if I feel sick with worry or sick from period pains.

Just feel dead. What the fuck. Can we really be this "unlucky"? It has been 7 years – an entire secondary education and still it hasn't worked? I'm just not sure I can bear it. Dread going to the loo just to see more.

And then it stopped. Just like that.

It seemed like an eternity but we finally got to the six-week scan (which the IVF clinic does). I thought I was going to throw up – not from anything pregnancy related (to be honest I really didn't feel pregnant and despite what everyone says, I didn't feel different at all, which made me more nervous that it wasn't real); but from panic that they might not find anything. What if there is no heartbeat and this has been just another cruel twist?

Up again on the bed. Weird black and white images which made no sense to me.   Then the most precious words in the world, "there's a heartbeat".

Relief, pure, absolute joy just floods through me. Then, "wait a minute". Oh for fuck's sake, "no, no, no, that's not fair".

"Er, there are actually two heartbeats". Que even more joy, it was literally like the orchestra had broken out – that is the most amazing thing she could have said. I look across at Jason. He is staring at the screen hard and has gone slightly pale. I just beam at him. Beam and beam and beam.

I'm not religious but every night I went to bed (lying on my left as apparently that helps things) I said thank you, thank you for letting me be pregnant for another day. I think I was in shock for the entire pregnancy, no matter how big I got I didn't trust it, didn't think it would last.

But I also made sure I kept true to my promises, I didn't rub my belly once (at least not in public – turns out some of the rubbing maybe because it is itchy but that still doesn't excuse it), I didn't complain about being pregnant - what was there to complain about, after the hell of the last 7 years I would have accepted anything but maybe as a small piece of karma, the pregnancy was fine (I took to eating through nausea) but most of all I just kept willing myself to get to the birth part and for them to be ok – just be alive and ok.

Thirty-six weeks later, after a small complication with pre-eclampsia and an emergency caesarean which I could actually feel some of but didn't care because what mattered more than anything in the world was that, identical twin girls were born, 30 seconds apart. Screaming their heads off and sounding like piglets. They were whisked off to the ICU. It may have been the drugs but I just knew they were going to be fine and they really were – just a little small and needing some extra care before being released into the big wide world. Every night since, every single night since, I pinch myself at how aboundingly lucky I am and how grateful I am.

I promised myself during those nightmare years that if, if I ever did manage to have a baby I would not be over-protective. Having yearned so long and so hard for something I didn't want that to impact them, I wanted the child to be carefree and happy. And they really are the happiest, most wonderful, gorgeous bundles of joy.

Letter of Advice to my pre-trying self

**The advice that I would have given myself at the beginning of the
process if I could have (and if I would have listened) :**

Dear Me, aged 30

You have always thought that hard work was all that was required. You
never give up. Ever. You think you can have it all. You are stubborn.

You are wrong to think you can have it all; certainly in the way you
currently think. But all those other "qualities" keep. They are who you
are and if you think you can change them you are wrong. If you want to
have children, and I know that you really, really do, more than anything in
the world; not as a platitude of what women as supposed to want at this
age but as an aching, visceral, biological, life-affirming need, then you
need to adjust your thinking and your priorities. Your strategy has to be
what you say it is.

First, you need to think about work/life balance. You need to be living a
healthier life, with more sleep (a lot more sleep, 5 hours is not enough,
neither is 6), less stress (that churning feeling in the pit of your stomach
about every meeting, call and aggressive work situation needs to go). You

are never going to be a slow down, yoga type, so do what you love and what you can lose yourself in (a good book or film, a run, sport), anything that will just take your mind off all this for a moment.

Second, you need to be kinder to yourself. You need to ask for help and seek support where you can – it is not weak to do so, it is required; you are going to need it. That can also mean letting yourself avoid people with children, saying no to holidays and events with lots of children if you can't face it. That is okay. Protect yourself and your mental well-being. This is tough enough as it is.

Third, have a structured plan: basic tests before you start trying, try for six months, see a fertility specialist, decide the things that need to change with your lifestyle and your diet and change them, have an end game plan (whether it be surrogacy or adoption or both).

Fourth, it's not all about you. He may not take the same approach to all this as you do but Jason does love you and does actually need your support, not bitter recrimination on a constant basis. You need to try and find the right words to help him understand and you need to stop and consider what he is going through. You also need to look at your actions. If you moan about something but still do it, Jason takes that as you wanting to do it on some level or at least accepting it. If you want something to change, you need to show that by your actions, not just your words.

Fifth, understand the statistics. This is a numbers game. Understand your own numbers (your AMH etc.) as well as the general population, and when it comes to it, the numbers of your clinic.

Sixth, trust your gut. If you think something sounds like bullshit it probably is. If you want to go for a long, exhausting run, go for a long, exhausting run.

Seventh, buy a solid punch bag or a lot of second-hand crockery. That anger and bitterness needs a channel.

Eighth, if anyone tells you, you just need to relax, you have my full permission to tell them to go fuck themselves. If they already have children, feel free to punch them as well (okay maybe not actually punch them but feel free to feel you want to).

Finally, I know you won't, so I don't really need to say this, but don't give up. Ever. Keep fighting and keep pushing. Don't let the doctors push you around. If one doctor isn't willing to help, find another one.

Take care and if things get really bad, please, please, get help. Any help, because there is always hope, no matter how bad it gets. There is always hope, so keep going.

A x

"This above all: to thine own self be true, and it must follow, as the night the day, thou canst not then be false to any man."

Polonius' speech in Hamlet by William Shakespeare

THE MALE PERSPECTIVE

1

Introduction (Or How Sex Isn't Always the Answer)

One day I was having dinner with my wife and she turned to me and said that she thought we should have lots more sex. I agreed with her, and all was good.

OK, the conversation was actually more like this:

She says, "I think we should try to have children."

I hear: "Let's have lots of sex."

I say, "Definitely!"

There was more discussion around it being a big responsibility, us having hit a certain point in our lives, and other such things, but frankly, I'm really just agreeing, I mean honestly, why wouldn't I?

Then I'm thinking, do we start now? It turns out that the answer is yes... I'm happy.

For several months this continues. We have more sex than we've had in a long time, I'm happy, and she's not happy. I mean, I think the sex is ok, but she's not pregnant. I blithely say, "Don't worry, we just need to keep going... how about now?"

I think this might have been the point where our paths diverged. At this point she thinks I'm just in it for the sex (I'm probably 90% in it for the sex, but I do want children too), and I haven't helped.

The sex changes. It becomes more... timed, managed, and she starts trying to make sure we're hitting ovulation, or 3 days before ovulation, or 2 days afterwards. Now is not a good time, now is. No, not now, your sperm won't be optimal because we had sex yesterday.

Now, I'm not complaining (much) but it's not entirely how I imagined things.

Here are a couple of scenarios I experienced:

First one - I was kicked awake (almost literally) by my wife. She looked exhausted, she'd just peed on a stick, and she said, "We have to do it now..." At this point I'd be thinking, this is good! Then she said, "But be quick, we only have 5 minutes because otherwise I'll miss my train." Um, what, I'm barely awake and you want me to... Yes, she did. Now I would get up and get to it, but it was not a huge amount of fun (though Blitz sex always had some appeal), and the constant "Hurry-ups!" didn't help. At the end I was left a little bit bruised (not quite literally), and then had to rush to shower, get dressed and leave to catch the same train.

Second one - "Damn, it's day 14!" I'd say to yourself, "I'm sure it's the 3rd." But I knew by now not to argue. She then says, "We have to have sex, but quickly, it's late and I have to get up early in the morning." This is a repeat of the morning one, but worse, because the deadline is arbitrary, and you're tired, I mean really, does it have to be right now? Can we not wait till the morning? No. Do it now.

I don't know, but I suspect these scenarios didn't do much for my sperm quality, but at the time that was not yet something I thought about.

She also started getting blood tests, and then she had an operation to check things were ok after being treated for endometriosis. Her uterus is described as pristine. What do you say to that? But it's all becoming a little more fraught, a little less lingerie and lubricant. Well to be honest there's more lubricant, but shiny machine oil more than scented luxuriant massage oil.

Sperm Test

Then one day she mentions I should have a sperm test. As I recall, it was in passing, in a sort of, just to make things are ok at your end kind of way. Almost as if she thought I would respond badly. She was right.

Really. I mean me, look at me, I'm the picture of slightly-overweight-ok-by-quite-a-bit-manliness, working like a dog, commuting two hours each way every day, and really not at all stressed. My sperm is going to be great, and I don't need some white coated authority to judge me.

I'm also, let's be honest here, a little nervous. I mean, what if my little swimmers aren't up to scratch. I have reason to think they might not be too, because when I was 5 I had an operation on an undescended testicle. It got stuck, it hurt, they fixed it, it involved knives and my scrotum, and I've got to think there's a risk they might not be great.

So I wuss out, I suggest that perhaps we just need to keep going, the stats say etc, etc.

This, it appears, is a mistake, because, now, not only am I obsessed with sex (I'm a man...) but I'm also not helping with the whole baby thing, I'm not even trying. Even worse, I don't realise that I'm implicitly blaming her. It is not at all clear to me, but this is the first, small, step in a new stressful direction.

By this point she's been seeing a slightly crazy Chinese woman who is trying to help, but mostly seems to end up upsetting my wife. Now she wants to see me as well, and then she wants me to do some tests. The first is a sperm test. The second is blood.

I'll come back to the blood, but I do agree to have the sperm test. This is in part because having a slightly manic traditional Chinese medical practitioner stare at you while you try and explain why it isn't such a great time... well it doesn't work. It's also because I've realised that I should do this test, it's important, because quite frankly if there is an issue then we need to know. More importantly, I don't like it when my wife goes into hospital and has general anaesthetics, it makes me nervous (hospitals were places where I visited people shortly before they died on a number of occasions when I was young), and it would appear that some of the next stages in the infertility "journey" will require more hospital visitations. If these are a waste of time, or something bad happens, and it turns out I could have avoided it by 'producing a sample', then I'd never forgive myself. So, I say yes, she gives me an impressive little form, which she ticks lots of boxes on.

I arrange my appointment. I'm not great on the phone at the best of times, and phoning up a posh sounding woman to arrange a... well anyway, I did it, blushing into the phone, and got a slot.

It's my first time, and so I check the instructions. One of the requirements is that I refrain from sex for at least three days. I jokingly mention that this isn't going to help in the production of babies to my wife. It seems she does not find this in the least amusing.

The location is near Harley Street, the buildings are impressive, and I walk into an atrium, with a severe looking couple of women at a desk. It's like they're making it difficult, but at least I don't have to say anything I just hand over my form, they look at it dismissively, and then tell me to wait in the waiting room. This is like a Victorian bric-a-brac shop. There are many sofas, which were nice once, and tables, and lampshades, all somewhat haphazardly strewn around the room. It is thankfully empty, though cold. I wait. A nurse comes in and calls my name, and she leads me to a tiny room.

The room is clean, and lacks windows, which is good. She explains the process, well, not the actual process, but the washing, and the writing on the form, and the noting the time and such like. I'm listening attentively but fail to really catch any of it because I'm trying to concentrate on not being embarrassed. Fortunately it's also all written down on the sheet of paper she gives me. I do not think I actually looked at her during the entire time she was talking to me.

There are some materials (at this clinic the materials are pretty good, at others... well...), as well as a plastic pot, and a piece of paper, and well, that's it. Some minutes later I have completed my task, filled in forms and signed them, and placed these all, contained in a plastic envelope, into an in-box on the way out. I was told I had to go back to the waiting room. So I did.

Then I'm called up again and told I need to give some blood, just a blood test, not pints or anything. I freak out. My excuse is that when I was 15 I passed out while having a blood test, and have had a phobia ever since. I'm unclear whether I knew I was supposed to do this, but I genuinely can't cope with it, and after a few minutes of trying the nurse gives up on me and sends me on my way. The look of contempt on her face haunted me for some time.

Ask any phlebotomist (blood sucker) and they'll tell you blokes are the worst, complete wusses in fact. But at this point I was secretly shamed, and didn't tell any of my friends about it.

This is strike two. I have refused to give a little blood, I mean really, am I trying to get her pregnant or what? (I am... I mean, I just assumed that, you know, all that was required was sex!).

My sperm by the way was good. Well... decent volume, and a high % of abnormalities, but not beyond the parameters. I felt vindicated. Or at least not emasculated. This is slightly different from my wife's recollection, but we both agree that there were no obvious red flags.

But now we're in a fix. She's got nothing wrong with her, and I'm fine (though could be better...). So what do we do?

It turns out the wrong answer is to suggest more sex.

At this point we're now on opposite sides, only, I don't realise that at the time. I'm still not getting this thing, and that's because I'm deaf to the giant clock which is ticking in my wife's head. Every minute of every day it's saying "Bay-bee... Bay-bee". I can't hear that. All I can hear is "sex?…tra la la…sex?…tra la la".

I'm thinking... I need to earn money, to pay the mortgage. Work is nightmarish, but if I put in a little more, I might get a promotion or a raise, or buy myself some breathing space. I'm thinking, it would be nice to have a break, go somewhere with my wife. Wait, what happened to my wife, she appears to have gone insane, and now, what, she really wants me to do a blood test?

Around this time I had to have a medical for insurance. The nurse came to my work and took my blood pressure. She said it was high and refused to tell me what it was, she told me to relax, and took it again, and then said she'd try again after the questions. She took it again, and said that while it would have no impact on my insurance I should go and see the doctor right away. I kind of felt a bit of tension was ok as the medical happened to be in the only free slot I had that day, and my next meeting was presenting to the boss, who wasn't always that forgiving.

But I went to the doctor's and my blood pressure was high, not crazy, but not safe. They asked me to come back a few days later, and suggested I avoid caffeine that morning, which I did, and they took my blood pressure again. This time they said I was just below the level at which I would have to start taking pills. One of the suggestions the nurse made was that I should get a home blood pressure tester. On the one hand I was concerned this might make me more stressed, but on the other hand I like data, so I got one, and my blood pressure at home was consistently lower than the measurements at the doctor's, or hospital for that matter. I have mild white coat syndrome it would seem…

It was shortly after this that I gave up caffeine, and was more or less caffeine free for seven years, at least in part because the two weeks of withdrawal headaches horrified me into keeping off it.

Scourges: Temperature Charts

Anyway, things were proceeding, or not proceeding. My months have several nightmare days, when her period comes. There is literally nothing I can say or do at this point which helps. Even a good bottle of wine doesn't help... her. But I think I'm probably drinking a bit more now. Just a little.

Two new things have entered our lives, temperature charts and mucus. I mean, the mucus was there before, and to be honest I rarely ever thought about it, but now it needs to be springy? Or something? Anyway, it's not a thing I've been equipped by life to discuss. But, occasionally its state is such that it means she's at a key fertile point in her cycle and we should have sex, which seems positive.

The temperature charts on the other hand are pure and utter evil. As soon as she wakes up she takes her temperature. This is then carefully noted down on a specific chart. Over the course of the month this temperature is intended to show where her menstrual cycle is, and... well I am not really sure about the 'and'. I guess it's supposed to help in timing sex, but honestly from all the anecdotal stories, it seems that it is possible for a woman to get pregnant at any stage in her cycle - yes I know, but women have become pregnant after having sex while menstruating, it's a thing. Anyway, my wife's cycle was not 'typical', meaning it wasn't a regular, clockwork 28 days. This may be common, but the literature is very fixed on 28 days to the extent that it provided almost no guidance at all for any other length of cycle.

So anyway, we now take note of the temperature, it's too high, it's too low, it's too similar to the previous day... But that's not all of it, because other things affect the temperature. How quickly after waking up it's taken (apparently). Or the time we went to bed. My wife worked (works) hard and so would often not come to bed until very late, and this of course meant she didn't get enough sleep, and then her temperature was 'wrong'. Some months, when work was particularly bad, the charts were literally all over the place. Flying and time zone changes also play havoc. All in all, it's a real challenge to get a good temperature chart. And when you do... well, nothing. It made no difference at all the few (very few in reality) times her charts were vaguely like the perfect examples. I tried very hard to see the positives in the charts, but even when they were unequivocally 'good', she didn't get pregnant.

That's why I think they're evil, because they really told us nothing useful, and all they did for us was ensure that my wife started worrying about babies right at the beginning of the day, and often would already have assumed the month was going badly before it was even clear that was the case. And even in the months when the chart was looking relatively 'normal' in the early stages, it didn't help pointing it out. All in all, they were truly horrible things which added to our general misery.

I suspect somebody is going to do some proper research and determine lots of useful things from all these charts, but until then I will maintain my hatred for them.

Challenges: Other Women Getting Pregnant

And what do I do when a friend tells me his wife is pregnant? If I tell her, it's bad, if I don't tell her and she finds out I knew and didn't tell her then it's worse. So I start to try and time these things... oh, a good temperature this morning, things are proceeding well, oh yes I must have forgotten Blahblah is pregnant. This doesn't always work, but it's better than the other way.

The other thing is that I start to notice pregnant women, and they're everywhere. My wife mentioned it, and I expressed some form of disbelief, but now, I can see them too; she's right. They're there. And do you know what they're doing, they're rubbing their bellies. Continuously. It seems to me that they're also looking around, trying to find the women who don't have babies, so they can rub their bellies at them... wait, no, it's not me who thinks that, it's the women trying to have a baby. I think they're just rubbing their bellies, because, they itch or something. Even so it is an odd phenomenon, which if you haven't noticed before, will now haunt you (you're welcome…).

There are also the baby on board signs. There are the ones which women wear on the underground to encourage others to give them seats. These rarely impact me as I always stand, partly because I read somewhere that standing is good for you, and partly to avoid the potential of having to actually communicate with someone about offering them a seat. It astonishes me in equal part how often people ignore the obvious needs of such women, and then how often someone will give up their seat, but only after half the journey has passed. It's like there's some kind of test, a certain time to wait to make sure the pregnant woman really needs the seat. If she's wearing the badge, then I figure she does, and if I was sitting I'd give her my seat (I have done so on the extremely rare times when I am both sitting and the need has arisen).

The other type is the one on cars. I really don't see the point of these. Is it supposed to encourage people to give them more space? I read a piece of research which implied that they were actually causing more accidents, partly because they reduced the driver's view, and partly because they were distracting when they moved about. Nonetheless, I put these in the bragging category. This can be shown by the many derivatives, princess on board, twins on board etc, etc. They're exactly as annoying as the stickers showing the family (which again are a boast, look how many children we have, and how individual we all are).

Those are my feelings. My wife's can only be described as terrible anger. The women on the tube she only hated a little bit, the cars brought out the kind of rage normally reserved for the idiot in the BMW 1-series who swings out of the feeder lane and cuts up three lanes of traffic.

Despite all this, I kept trying to make it sound like it was all going to be ok, but she didn't believe me. I think the problem is partly the statistics. If some doctor (or IVF clinic brochure) says 1 in 3 women will get pregnant this year, and I see a pregnant woman, does that mean my wife is not going to get pregnant, if I see, say, a dozen in the local area does that mean we should give up entirely? Or move to a less fertile area, except wouldn't that be the wrong answer? I'm thinking this, and I know she is, and it's crazy. We've entered an unhappy twilight world of madness, a purgatory where we get to roll the dice every month, and hopefully, this month, we'll win the jackpot. Except we aren't. And the months pile up.

We heard a lot about the cliff at forty, how a woman's fertility nose-dives. I'll be honest, I always found this irritating. It's not entirely clear what we're supposed to do with the information, and given that two-thirds of infertility cases are officially 'unexplained' (this is something we were not told until round 3 of our IVF journey) it seems odd that there can be such certainty in a different part of the spectrum. I realise there are lots of statistics out there, but given the general dearth of data on women's bodies, cycles etc, it seems like there might be a bunch of reasons for it which bear investigating and which might not apply. I think it's an easy excuse, and it needs to be properly tested.

Nonetheless, it's there, and it tends to overshadow things, it tends to make women feel like there is a ticking time-bomb, and they need to get moving or it'll be too late, and if only we'd started when I wanted to...

It also seems to be the case that male fertility does not follow such a cliff, though poorer sperm quality definitely comes with age, and this may also impact children (though the science is, unsurprisingly, mixed on this as well). This creates another gap between partners, another point of contention, which is genuinely unhelpful.

This general state of purgatory might have gone on for a while, but for the fact that we earned enough money to consider a medical solution. In Virto Fertilisation - IVF.

2

IVF (No Sex Required)

So IVF. It's this thing where, well, you know, test-tubes and whatnot. In our entire time of trying I never saw anything which looked like a test-tube. It was rather disappointing.

The thing with IVF is when you start you assume it's a big thing. We went to a doctor on Harley St (we wanted the best... more fool us). He said we were going to do a 'diagnostic' IVF, which would tell us where the problem was.

In retrospect, this was not entirely true. He was just a salesman. IVF is an industry, and I wished I'd known that at the beginning, because we would not have gone with him. Or the next people for that matter. But I didn't, so...

One of the things he said was that we should keep having sex (I liked him for that), as for many people just starting the IVF cycle was enough to produce pregnancy, he even named a practice who had more success on their waiting list than in the actual procedures. I should have probably thought that through a bit more, but he'd at least given me the green light. I'd also had to have another sperm test (same place, materials still good). At our next appointment with the test results he said my sperm was perfect. Perfect. Ha.

My wife and I disagree on what happened for this cycle. As I recall, I went to a number, though not all, of the preparatory meetings. And while I did not administer the injections (in my memory this was because she thought I'd be inept enough to cause her some pain because I had the blood phobia, she may have been right), I did mix the drugs and help monitor it. More importantly, or at least more prominent in my memory, I had a blood test for the first time in at least 15 years.

The law requires a blood test to check for diseases before an IVF cycle, so there were no possible arguments. So I traipsed off to the lab to have it, my wife at my side, to support me, and quite possibly drag me to the needle if required. I was very lucky, the nurse was lovely, when I explained what a wuss I was, somewhat sheepishly, she said that she too had problems giving blood, made sure I could lie down, talked to me all the way through and even brought me some Lucozade afterwards. She was amazing. My wife was grudgingly impressed that I didn't faint away. Fortunately, the results came through all fine.

I have since had blood tests from nurses and phlebotomists who appear to delight in tormenting men who have a blood test phobia. In addition, my arms are quite hairy, and they, for some reason, have to find the biggest, stickiest plaster in the world. I swear it hurts more than the blood test itself. I am extremely grateful to that first nurse, otherwise I might have run away...

During the sales pitch it's never mentioned that IVF is a really tough process. For the woman. For the man it might be as little as turning up for one quick session in a clinic to produce a small vial of swimmers which will be expertly mixed with some eggs - which are extracted in a much more invasive process. For the woman it's not just the injections, the egg collection, and the (if there are good enough options) reintroduction of the potential future embryos. It's that the drugs they are pumping themselves with (unless their partner is capable and trusted to inject) are hormones, which directly affect their emotions and mood, but in much greater quantities than usual. And I'll be honest, I didn't make any allowance for it that first time (or the second really), so well, let's say I did not earn any brownie points. Actually, all I remember is being knackered from work, being in the middle of trying to get to appointments (which at this point were all in London and literally hours away from work), and being in the dog house no matter what I did. Maybe if I'd thought it through... but I didn't. If I do discover a time machine in the future, I'm still going to write this paragraph, but I'm going to make sure that neither my wife nor I actually have to live through the whole experience again.

One of the things which made both our lives more difficult was that hospital planners are either incompetent or insensitive (or evil, but I'll discount that). For every process involved we had to walk through the maternity ward. Yes, here we were, trying hard to make a child happen, and we get to see the outcome (which if you've ever been in one of those wards you'll know isn't quite sunshine and frolics with screaming babies and exhausted mothers all around but still). For me it was an irritant, for her it was yet more salt. I did read at some point that women who want to have children should spend a lot of time with pregnant women, as there's some kind of hormonal transference or whatever, but I'm not entirely convinced the mental side would make it worth it.

Other clinics have many, many pictures of their IVF babies. This is also in somewhat poor taste.

The first IVF didn't work. The reason given was… we were just unlucky, and we should do another one. No diagnostics, no data, no nothing.

Let down by that first doctor, we decided to have the second IVF at a different industrial complex. We were promised much more data. The cycle was not successful. Worse there was no data, what we received was an "oh well, nothing obvious wrong, here's the prescription for the next round", or, to paraphrase "give me another 5.5k and you can roll the dice again".

We had a rethink. Actually, we didn't. We really should have.

We went for a third roll of the dice, but this one was on the NHS, based on some weird local logic which meant that we were eligible but only within a surprisingly tight window before the rules were going to change and we'd be out of luck. I'll admit to being happy that we were going to be spending someone else's money (well I guess technically our tax money) on the dice roll.

This time my sperm was not up to scratch. This was a kick to the metaphoricals. They don't really know why sperm samples vary so much (and they do vary, lots more than you might be led to believe), but I'll be honest, I'm fairly certain I know what the problem was, it was the room I had to use to produce the 'sample'. It was opposite the nurses' coffee room. Now maybe you're thinking, nurses, uniforms, that's pretty sexy, you should have been well up for it. Instead you should be thinking, three women, chattering loudly about their day, their patients, etc, knowing that you are there, probably 10ft away, currently trying to produce a sample courtesy of some shiny pictures of Sharon from Kent, but doing so in the approved manner per the poster on the wall (sample production should take 15 minutes, you should clean everything, ensure you get the entire sample into the container, which means taking the lid off first, but don't get anything contaminating in it, look Sharon, just wait a moment, I'm reading the next bit, oh yes, note the time the sample was produced, right, and then... did I wash my hands, yes, right, let's go..), and in background, coffee being made, chit chat, and giggles, which aren't at all coquettish. Anyway, I was a true hero, and produced my sample. And it was criticised.

This time it had to be ICSI. This is the same process as for a standard IVF, but instead of just mixing the sperm and ova together and shaking (they might not actually shake them), the sperm are individually selected and introduced to the ova. It's the difference between speed dating and arranged marriage (possibly). ICSI costs more, but as we weren't paying this time it wasn't a concern for me. I don't think my wife would have cared either way.

I do wonder though, if we were paying, would it be a real question, I mean could I have said "No dear, this joyous process is already costing us 5k, I refuse to pay another 700 quid so some technician can pick through my sperm to select the ones which don't have two tails and can actually swim." It felt like it wouldn't go well. It's another part of the industrial side I didn't like, not least as the clinic is the one which decides if ICSI is the right answer.

Anyway, after all of that, including another session opposite the nurses' coffee room, the cycle didn't work either. In the sense that my wife was not pregnant at the end of the process. However we had produced enough high quality blastocysts and morulas that we could put them on ice. Yay. This of course cost extra money, which we had to pay for this time. I think this was worth it, as it gave us some hope, we'd actually managed to get further down the line and produce more and better – perhaps ICSI was the answer? It also would have been difficult, perhaps impossible, to just throw those potentials away, which was the other option.

So, if we wanted to take another shot, we could go through half the process, basically the hormone stuff for my wife, and then implantation, no extraction of ova, or sample production, it sounded a little less stressful. The doctor helpfully told us that you know, maybe we were just unlucky, and that what we had was 'unexplained' infertility, which affects two-thirds of cases, and maybe we should just consider adoption (or my wife should relax - she still gets angry when I suggest she relax). This also did not go down well with me. Firstly, I wasn't ready to consider adoption, I felt we were giving up early, but secondly, two-thirds unexplained? What the actual. The confident sales, the smiles and nods of encouragement, all from people (professionals, medical, highly trained, allegedly scientific, professionals) who did not know what was going on two thirds of the time. I was genuinely incandescent.

I have since come to the conclusion that this is for two major reasons. Number 1, IVF works, often, and it produces lots of money, so, sure, work on making IVF better, but replace it? (Cynical, I know.)

Secondly, it is flabbergasting how little medical research is done involving women, let alone women trying to get pregnant. It is about as close to zero as it's possible to get, in fact, it's a genuine miracle they even got as far as working out IVF. Read the excellent book 'Invisible Women' by Caroline Criado-Perez if you want to know more on this.

Anyway, there we were, and that was it, I had had enough. It was time to take charge. I wanted answers, and I wanted a plan.

So I suggested that I be in charge of the process for a year.

My initial plan was to take 6 months off, go to various holiday spots and shag like rabbits, but... a combination of mortgage, fear of having to find a new job, and the even bigger fear that my wife might actually explode if I suggested such a thing, made me come up with a different plan. I still think that first plan would've worked...

I wanted more data, and I wanted to approach it as a process.

Therefore, we did a bunch more tests. We spoke to some more people, and we planned. We also lost weight (quite a lot in my case) and got a lot fitter. And drank less alcohol, though not nothing. We also tried to reduce the work stress in our lives, with some limited success.

One of the people we spoke to was a doctor in the US who specialised in helping people get pregnant without using IVF. He was a former IVF practitioner who'd become a little cynical about the process. We had a conference call and he was great. He confirmed that we were doing a number of the right things, he suggested we eat healthily and all of that good stuff. He also made two suggestions which I followed immediately, one was to stop having my mobile phone in my front pocket. I'm not sure if this was to do with the transmission of radio waves or the potential heating effect, but I made the change, and have never reverted. The other was that I stop having hot baths. This was hard for me, I love a big hot bath, relaxing with, and this was also frowned upon, a large glass of red wine. Bliss. Gone. But this was important, nobody, in 6 years, had ever mentioned these things. I was feeling justified in our new approach.

Some of these tests we'd done before, but here's where we became a little more focused, and actually understood a little more of what they meant. Things like AMH levels, and overall sperm health are important to know.

There's loads of tests which can be done, and I recommend to anyone who's willing to spend 5k on IVF, to first spend 1-2k on as many tests as possible. Blood tests (general and fertility specific), general health tests, and specific investigations. These may save you a tremendous amount of stress and grief, and will give you an idea of where you stand.

I had to give blood several times during this period. I believe I was getting better at it. Here's a tip though...

While most of the time the person taking your blood will be a nurse, and therefore statistically likely to be female, it's best not to presume.

I have a friend who had to have a series of blood tests. On one occasion a woman entered into the cubicle to take his blood and he said, "Oh thank God, a nurse. Doctors are always terrible at blood tests." She was the doctor. It has never hurt more.

Though he was right, doctors do tend to be worse, less practice mainly. So, if you have a choice, the order is phlebotomist, nurse and then doctor. And never ever insult, or risk insulting, someone who is about to stick something sharp into you.

Also, if you think you might pass out, tell them. They think you're a wimp already, and they'd rather have you on the bed, than slumped on the floor with a head wound (almost a word for word quote from one of the nurses).

In my case there were also two specific tests which are worth recounting, though for different reasons.

The first was a special sperm test called a sperm fragmentation test, which was performed at the same clinic as my very first test. (I think by the end I'd produced samples there six or seven times). Anyway, this test is very specific, and costs about 500 quid. We decided that it was worth doing, I book the test and I trotted off to the clinic confidently, I knew the drill now. Checked out the materials, all pretty good, and the room is comfortable, and either specially acoustically insulated or at least in a very low noise space, so no risk of being disturbed. I perform my function, and I'm pretty happy with what I've produced. I write down the times and take my sample with me.

Now different places have different processes, my favourite was the one where you just put it into a cupboard in the wall, and the lab could take it out from the other side. Very discrete. This place, well, I was told to put it on the table in the entrance to the lab. After my sample production I walked in, just wanting to deliver it and go, and I was stopped by a tall female nurse, who checked my piece of paper. She then picked up the sample and peered at it. I'm feeling uncomfortable now. After a pause she says, in a strong German accent, "I don't think this will be enough," and gives me the evil eye. I'm stutteringly proposing to go back into the room to produce more, when she clucks and says she'll check it, whereupon she takes my sample and puts it on some kind of super weighing machine which bips and beeps away. She scowls at the result, returns to me, and says, "It's only just enough." With that I'm dismissed, and I leave the lab with my tail between my legs.

The only positive out of the experience was that the result came back fine, which was good because I think if the answer had been a no then we'd have been out of luck. The downside of course is it didn't help get any closer to determining the unexplained nature of our situation.

The other test I had was an ultrasound check on my testicles. We had heard via one of my wife's friends of a thing called varicoceles, which are basically where the veins in a man's testicles get a little blocked and start to swell. It's the testicular equivalent of varicose veins. Googling it was instructive, though the images were slightly disturbing. Anyway, there is a theory that this may have an impact on male fertility but the science is, once again, surprisingly light on the ground. Her friend's husband had visited a doctor in Israel to get it fixed.

One of the things I'd decided on when starting the year of being in charge was that we would try, as much as possible, things which would improve our chances. Anything which gave just a small percentage improvement was worth doing.

This being the plan, I went to a private clinic to have the ultrasound. I believe it was not possible to have it done on the NHS unless there were obvious signs, such as bulging testicles and discomfort, but varicoceles can be reasonably large without causing either of these. I swear I was told by the nurse to take my boxer shorts off and lie on my front, so I did. I was nearly asleep when the ultrasound woman came in. She seemed quite disconcerted, but once I was in the right position she got to work. I'll be honest, paying a woman a lot of money to rub gel onto my testicles and take pictures had always in my mind been a very different and far more enjoyable experience.

The results were that I had varicoceles, one in each testicle. This was a victory! An actual thing we could do something about, and finally something demonstrably wrong with me, and possible cause of the occasional bad sperm test such as the one which led to the ICSI round. Yay. What do we do?

There are a couple of methods of dealing with it, but basically it is performed by a radiologist who cuts into a vein and feeds a camera and tube into you and then finds the testicle, implants a sort of metallic umbrella thingy which blocks the bad vein and you're done. Sadly, no trip to Israel for me, it turned out it was possible to get the procedure done at our local hospital.

When I met with the radiologist he asked me why I was doing it, and I told him about our desire to have children, and that I'd heard it might have an impact. He was surprised, and clearly exasperated, that I'd had to hear a story third hand before I had even known to check for it, and he asked me to tell him the results of our next IVF (or if we had children naturally) as he was trying to gather evidence to support a proper study into varicoceles and their impact.

Weirdly my private health wouldn't pay for it, but the NHS would, and given it was to be done in the same hospital by the same people this didn't seem to be a problem, I just had to wait an extra month. This was fine.

Of all the various things we did over those years this particular procedure was the most embarrassing, and oddly I can't explain why. It was just surreal, and a bit uncomfortable.

I'm prepped, which basically means I am naked under one of those silly gowns and I've had some water. A nurse then led me to the theatre, where I got onto the bed, which is raised up. Another nurse then lifts up the front of the gown, puts something flat hard and cold over my groin and pushed down. Hard. She then lowers the scanner machine, presses again. I'm now set up. The radiologist comes in, he's very nice, a bit chatty, dabs my neck, cuts it and starts feeding in the cable. This felt extremely odd. Cold and then, well just odd. He's assisted by the first nurse, who is making sure that everything feeds through properly. It's at this point that I notice a third woman, who is standing and watching. I have no idea who she was or why she was there, I don't believe she was introduced, but she made the process even more weird.

The radiologist very quickly finds the entrance to my left testicle, deploys the umbrella thingy, which would have been more exciting if it hadn't also required further pressure on my groin. Did she have to push down so hard? Anyway, then we start looking for the entrance to my right testicle, I say "we" because I felt part of the team at this point. Minutes drag by, the process is described in somewhat wearied terms as 'tiresome' by the radiologist and I'm starting to worry, I mean, I'm here, I'm ready, I'm spread out and you know, I don't think I can be any more open, so, please don't tell me you can't do it...

He couldn't. After nearly 40 minutes of looking for my right testicle he apologised and gave up. Apparently, the entrance to the left is easy to find and the right is always tricky. I have reason to believe (as a result of that childhood undescended testicle) that my system is perhaps even more complicated, but there it was, a partial success. It was clear that there would be no further attempt.

Still, I felt that this was positive, I'd improved at least one of my testicles. It was time to roll the dice again.

It was at this point that my mother gave us a CD of pan pipes to play... it was never clear when she expected us to play them, but anyway, they were apparently very effective for the whole fertility thing. We still have that CD. It is still in its wrapper...

I'm going to step away from my side of the story at this point. The next two sections are written with hindsight. If I could go back and slap myself I would, but I can't. Here's what I would have told myself had I been able.

First things first, you need to understand the priorities.

Priorities

In the middle of something which has gone on for years, has no real end in sight, and is becoming more and more stressful, it is important to have priorities. Even more important is to know what your partner's priorities are.

Here is a rough list of my priorities, starting with a top 5. The order of these may have switched a little from time to time but it's more or less representative of what was worrying me.

My Number 1 - Work

My work was (and in a lot of ways still is) very important to me. It was also very stressful, time consuming and probably health damaging. I committed a lot of time and emotional energy to it, and it paid well. I was concerned about keeping my job in the ups and downs, I wanted to get paid more, and I wanted to get promoted. I wanted to do well at work, and be able to pay for nice things, and live well.

My job also involved travel for quite a while, which was useful for meeting people, and helping further my career, well at least I thought it was. However, it is rather difficult to procreate at transatlantic distances.

It was rare that this was not my number one priority.

Her Number 1 - Babies

She wants a baby. She wants one now.

My Number 2 - Money

I worry about money quite a bit. Possibly because of the lack of money when I was growing up, and possibly because we're constantly over-committing (mortgage, renovations, holidays etc). In fact, we are, despite earning a decent amount of money, in quite a bit of debt.

This means that I track it, make sure we are saving some just in case we have a real crisis, keep an eye on the credit cards, and move them when rates change, and generally worry. It takes time, and emotional energy.

Her Number 2 - Babies

She wants a baby. Immediately.

My Number 3 - My wife

I want my wife to be happy. I love her very much, and her happiness and well-being are very important to me. If I could give her a baby immediately I would. I'm trying, I really am.

Her Number 3 - Babies

She wants a baby. Why hasn't one appeared?

My Number 4 - Babies

I'd like to have children, a legacy, a happy wife (ok this is a follow on from 3), and to do so before I'm Charlie Chaplin's age (not now, when he had his last one). This is real, I'm not just saying this because my wife wants babies. I see friends starting to have kids and I'm jealous, I just didn't realise it would be quite this hard.

Her Number 4 - Babies

She wants a baby. Why is it so difficult?

My Number 5 - Friends

I moved around a lot as a child, and so I tend to hold on to my friends. They're important to me. This means I like to see them, either visit them wherever they live, or have them come and visit us. As everyone seems to move around a lot these days it's a bit harder than it used to be.

169

The downside of this is that it often involves alcohol, which continues to be a bone of contention.

Her Number 5 - Rural poverty in Patagonia

No, sadly, it's babies. She wants to have a baby.

The problem is, I didn't know this AT THE TIME. AT ALL. In fact, I've only really understood the full picture while we've been writing this book.

It led to a gap which added so much stress to our lives. I assumed that because she was doing all these other things (work, sport, friends etc.) it meant that having a baby, while obviously important, wasn't the only priority. In retrospect if I'd understood then we would have made some different decisions, and done so much earlier on. Your partner may not be able to articulate this. She might not be rocking in a corner. She might even be occasionally flippant. But I guarantee, based not just on my wife, but others I have spoken to, she's only thinking about one thing, and she only has one priority.

My other priorities...

During this period **my father** became ill and died. It was obviously a difficult time for me, and I handled it in my usual way, by burying it and trying not to worry about it. I also had to make sure my mother was OK, and support her, I didn't have a lot left over for my wife. Even so my wife was amazing during the whole of it, she handled lots of the painful admin and general mess, she was brilliant. But, even through all of it, she had one priority, babies. This was not obvious to me.

Animal husbandry. While doing all of this, we had a sort of small holding.

It was an adventure we'd started together, first with two goats we saved from ending up as curry, and they were followed by poultry, sheep, pigs, cows and alpacas... but all of these consumed a lot of time, energy and money. At certain times of the year, lambing, summer showers, and when the water pipes froze, they became an important priority. In addition, whenever we were in an IVF cycle, and my wife was injecting herself with all the hormones and suchlike, or at times when I was using various chemicals, she wasn't able to help me. Something which had started out as a joint mad project, became more and more mine, and I missed her help, and she missed the fun bits (though I do wonder if she deliberately avoided some of the bits involving poo).

3

What Does Success Look Like?

This is the advice I'd have given myself right at the beginning of the process, if I could have.

For many men success is generally based around money and status. This is a good thing. It drives us forward. This status typically includes a lovely wife and 2.4 children, a house in suburbia and the Fonze living above the garage (I may have got a bit lost there). But the assumption is that it will come along naturally in due course as a reward for all the hard work, and all will be well. This can be the case... but you wouldn't be reading this book if it was.

This is an opportunity, genuinely, to stop and consider whether this stereotypical success is desirable. Or is it we've just been sold on it for so long we believe? I don't think it really matters if it is or not, I think the key is more to ask the question, because the answer may be that you, and your wife, want something different.

Fundamentally your lives will change when, if, you have children, and to be honest, if you're trying to have children and heading down the IVF route. It is far better to be consciously in control of this process then to drift along as I did.

The first thing is to work out what success looks like. When we were first married my wife and I talked about having four kids, we even had names for them (two boys and two girls, atypical names, each one about 18 months apart for a nice spread of ages). This was a little woolly, but more than many of my friends. Indeed I have friends, more than one set, who got married, and only then discovered that one partner really didn't want children, and the other really did. In some cases a compromise was found, and in others divorce ensued.

So, ask yourself, and your wife:

1) How many children?

2) Are you living in the right place for them?

3) What sort of life will you lead after they're born, will your wife look after them full time, will you, will you split it or will childcare be involved.

This is a form of visualisation, (i.e. imagine the thing you want, and it will come), but it'll also help you get engaged in the process, and provide something doable for you to do to show support to your wife.

1) How many children?

It seems ridiculous to ask this question if you have none, but there are many people who have fixed number in mind, and you may find you spend several years producing one and being content with that. You might assume that the madness is over, and then your partner is immediately planning the next, and the stress starts again. Or she might be overjoyed with one and not want any more, and you've always wanted half a dozen and she utterly refuses to start the madness again. Knowing this beforehand may help you in planning.

Note: If you only want one, and he or she arrives, you might also want to consider taking specific precautions to prevent more (the snip). I know of a couple who had twins, were very happy, didn't want any more, six months later she was pregnant... with triplets.

2) Are you living in the right place?

There are two aspects to this, one is pure practicality, and the other is about nesting.

Pure practicality first... if you live in a studio flat in the centre of London, this may present additional challenges when (if) a baby arrives. It might also be in a difficult location if you choose to have IVF given the travelling and general logistics. It might also add stress into your life (late night noises, too easy to go the pub). It is worth stepping back and looking for where you might live with a baby. Not least as house hunting can be fun. You can visit new places, try out new restaurants, and it's something you can do with your partner, think weekends away in the

Cotswolds. It will demonstrate another type of commitment to the endeavour (though in bad months it may also be worth skipping a weekend or two of house hunting).

In addition, there are a surprising number of people who only realise their flat is impractical for children after the baby was born, and moving to a new house with a young baby is an extraordinarily stressful thing to do. Worse if it's not immediately possible due to money or work commitments. Nine months sounds like a lot of time to get prepared, but it flies by, even if you get a full nine months of warning.

Nesting... Some people believe that in order for a woman to become pregnant she needs a comfortable and nurturing home, a nest. I'm mildly sceptical about this, but on the other hand, if your house is a wreck, the plumbing leaks, the electricity sparks and the only procreation occurring is the family of rats under the floorboards, the additional stress will definitely not be helping. Stress control is one of the most important things to consider, for both of you.

Making it about her (as long as you do so in a positive way) will also give her back some control which she will be really missing.

3) What will your life be like?

A bit like the first question, this seems presumptuous. But it's worth considering, planning and talking about. It may be that your job will cover all the costs and your wife taking five years off will have no impact on your plans for that holiday home in the Canaries. But it might also be that she earns a substantial chunk of the family income. I know I was worried about what might happen to the money when (if) we had children. This was bad as I let it eat away subtly at the back of my mind, so when I finally broached the subject it went badly as she had no idea I'd even been thinking about it. Finances are a tremendous source of tension in most people's lives, having a plan will mean you can shake out all of the conflict, or at least most of it, before it becomes a BIG THING.

If your parents or in-laws are around they might be able to help with childcare, but it is always sensible to ask the question, as a lot of people are happy to do a day or so now and again, but don't necessarily want to be tied down to one or more days every week (they need to get to their holiday home in the Canaries). You might be jaded in your job, I was, and the idea of taking a year off to deal with baby poo might seem attractive (I was shovelling so much shit at work through much of this period that nappies did seem bizarrely attractive). Your partner might well be outraged if you take the traditional stance and assume she'll stay at home, or if you assume that she'll go back to work. Talking about it, planning it, and knowing what you want will create a better environment.

Here's my idea of success:

Four children.

I look after them for a couple of years, then my wife takes over (and works part time) and I go back to full time.

We live in a big house in the country with a garden and maybe some chickens.

Then we retire somewhere warm.

One friend's idea of success is:

One child.

Wife looks after child until they leave home.

Nice house in zone 1-2 of London (outside space would be a bonus).

Another friend:

No children.

Wife works.

Flat in New York. Lots of partying.

(This one probably needs to have an honest conversation with his wife.)

You can add touches in... for example I really wanted to have a dog, a Labrador in fact. This couldn't happen while we lived in a small flat in the city and worked 80-hour weeks, so as part of moving out, I added the dog into the picture. Being near the in-laws can be a mixed blessing depending on how well you get on with them, but it may be part of your

177

partner's version of success. It's also reasonable to assume that grand-parents will want to be around quite a bit when babies arrive.

Once you've identified what success looks like, you can start planning for it, and putting a structure in place which helps you both feel like you're making concrete steps. Buying a new house takes time, and may require saving (and spending less on alcohol could help in several ways, as long as you don't head towards White Lightning). It's also a good plan to start to save money for the time when one or other of you aren't working.

Now you have a goal, your definition of success, you need a plan, you need to know what the steps along the way should be, and how you can make sure you have a chance of attaining your goal.

4

The Plan

This is the result of 20/20 hindsight and may initially seem impractical, but I strongly believe that it is the best way. There is a lot of anecdotal evidence to support what I'm suggesting, but not as much science (see previous comments on unexplained infertility). I've tried to consider all of the issues we faced and suggest a plan which I should have followed.

To reiterate, the most important piece advice I can give is that you need to realise your old life is over. She wants to have a baby, and that means now, and that means it all changes. It's not a case of try and fit in a few more months of clubbing and all-nighters (work or partying) before responsibilities of the baby mean you can't. It's done... you might give yourself one last big night, but after that, you need to commit.

You can still go out with your mates... but maybe only a couple of times a month. And not all night. And not to the point of utter inebriation.

Secondly, and fundamentally, you both need to acknowledge that this is a marathon, not a sprint, and realising this will ensure you get to the end in one piece (though it doesn't guarantee victory).

A lot of this advice costs money. Not all of it, but a lot. I think this was one of the hardest things for me to accept, I was extremely money conscious when we started (I'm a bit more relaxed these days – no, I'm not really, I just like to think I am), and was rather penny-wise. At the very least you need to accept you're going to have to spend money, and that means you need to start saving now. If (when) you have children, they are not cheap (though for a while at least you might be saving money by going out less), so getting some discipline on the finances won't hurt.

This is a multi-step plan, but you need to agree all of these steps up front, including stage 3. It may well be hard, and you might need to compromise, but it will be better in the long term, trust me. In addition, you absolutely need to be planning the sex side, to make it work for both of you, be fun, and be at the right time! You have a goal, and getting the sex right is a critical part of achieving that goal.

Stage 1 - Natural Process

This stage is all about doing the most you can to get your partner pregnant by natural means. This involves creating a plan which has three main parts: relaxation, tests and health, and sex.

Relaxation:

Your partner needs to take a break from the crazy, busy, super stressy, continuously mad life she has. Even if you think she has an easy time of it, there will be parts of her life creating tension and causing angst, and these need to be minimised.

This is important. If she's working and playing hard, she's not relaxing, she's not nurturing herself, and she's going to be stressing her system. Almost every doctor agrees that this will negatively impact her fertility, but as with everything else, we don't know by how much.

If possible, she should take a year's sabbatical from work. If a whole year isn't possible, as much as is. Or she might even want to reconsider her entire work life, either working from home, or even what job she should be doing. Yes, I know it sounds crazy, but are you serious about this? Work for most of us is draining at the very least. Imagine how much more relaxed she'd be if she wasn't getting up every morning, dealing with her manager or worrying about what her colleagues are doing.

She should stop doing the daily measuring (it's only going to be stressing her out). You should have some chilled out breaks away (preferably at peak fertility times), you need to look after her, and she needs to look after herself. No alarm clocks waking her up at 0600. Relaxation is the key. Catching up on some books, binge-watching Netflix. She might consider taking up crochet (or macramé), whatever it takes to get her off the ridiculous hamster wheel we all build for ourselves. No, that was actually my mother's suggestion which was absolutely not going to happen but the point is valid – to find something that she finds relaxing and then work out how to find the time for her to do it.

You need to minimise stress in her life, so, you worry about the money, about the bills, about anything you can. Other things which might help her and which would be worth talking about would include:

- A cleaner - a nice tidy house, and less housework, is often worth having (even if she isn't working!).

- Spa days, massages, a hot tub - not right for everyone this is true, but some people love them, and if your partner is one of these then you should prioritise. Not all the time, but maybe at critical times of the month.

- An exercise machine - running machines, free weights, yes she could go to the gym, but it's a chore to get there, it's full of people, the machines are never free, or are covered in other people's sweat, and having the ability to exercise in the home is a little luxury she might appreciate. On the other hand, she probably shouldn't take up triathlon training...

- Acupuncture - this has been shown to have some impact on fertility and some clinics now include this in IVF cycles, it might be worth considering as part of the natural stage too. Some people find it very relaxing, though personally the idea of lying still while someone stabs me multiple times with pins seems more like a nightmare.

- Life coach, psychiatrist, counsellor - this is a personal decision, but it's worth considering, sometimes speaking to someone else about the problem helps with perspective. Doing this in the early days might resolve potential conflict before it builds into something horrible.

Part of her stress will almost certainly be your stress. If your job consists of long hours, hard work and a tense environment, it's likely to spill onto her, even if only because you're grumpy after a long day at work and you don't really want to deal with another problem. You might want to consider if your job is right for you - yes I know this is even more crazy, because it'll all cost money, but you're only young once. If you moved to a new company or role at a more junior level for a year, would that really hurt your long term career (I'd suggest the opposite based on personal experience and anecdotal evidence, but this is not about career advice). You need to work out how you can relax as well, because this is a long-term thing.

Testing

Overall Medical Tests - If you haven't already you should both do some medical tests. There are companies who will take blood tests, check your liver function and give you an overall health check. Some do specific fertility tests as well, both for women, checking her AMH levels and all the various other indicators, and for men. It might also show that there are other health related things which need to be worked on, knowing these early will give you more of a chance to get them sorted (and in my case, unrelatedly, identify a genetic condition which needed urgent treatment!).

Sperm Test - definitely. In fact, I'd suggest several over the next few months. Sperm quality varies, and it's worth getting an idea of how much your sperm is changing. You also need to be aware that if you're stressed or there are unwelcome distractions it might impact what you produce, and you should probably try a test at a different place. There are a few different things they can test sperm for such as motility, total number, how many are deformed, if at all possible get everything checked. There are also genetic and fragmentation tests which can be done on sperm.

Self Tests – Think about how you feel, do things ache, are there odd pains. Maybe check for varicoceles, or check the symptoms. The more information you have, the more you can push the %s, even if it's only one or two points.

AMH (anti-Müllerian hormone) – for her

This is a key hormone which can give a reasonable proxy view of a woman's fertility, as it gives a guide to the number of eggs she has left. 3 or more is good. Less than that it's starting to be an issue. This should be one of the key things you have tested, preferably early on in the process.

This is just the start of the medical things we learned about, but slowly. I wish at the beginning I'd made a list, and been able to monitor the various things, and tick off the steps to check them.

Lifestyle

Review your lifestyle as well. Health and fitness should be considered critically. If you're not eating well, and are a little overweight, then look at improving your diet, getting some exercise in and losing a bit of weight. It will be amazing how much better you feel, and it'll improve your percentages.

Drink less alcohol, try to stop smoking, avoid refined sugar, you know all the things the doctor would tell you to do... only you need to do at least some of them. The health of you and your partner will impact your chance of conceiving, so everything you can do to improve it is worth it.

Other random things which are worth considering... no hot baths. Less (no) cycling. Move your mobile phone to your back pocket. Don't put a laptop on your lap. Looser underwear. In fact, make sure your testicles remain cool and unhindered at all times. That's an image I didn't need, but really, it is important, they are important, so protect them. They hang out externally for a reason – they need to be cool.

This is the most important aspect of the 'natural' phase, as this is where you can find out about yourselves, and any potential medical issues without being under the pressure of the IVF industry. And things might be revealed, you might have varicoceles, she might have endometriosis, if they do happen then you can do something about them, and you'll be in a better position to go forward.

Sex

For this part of the process you need to be having sex. Regularly, but not too frequently, multiple times a day may well be fun, but your sperm quality will nose-dive. Once every two/three days was the recommendation when we were trying.

Importantly, make it fun, enjoy it, but don't lose sight of the target (blow jobs won't get her pregnant, well, probably not). Urgent sex, the "we have three minutes to do this otherwise we'll miss the fertility window" kind, may make for a good story if it works, but I suspect it's rare. Plan it out, give yourselves time and space to do it properly.

I believe that good sex, which is enjoyed by both partners, and which takes a reasonable length of time is most likely to be successful. This is partly based on the signs at some clinics suggesting sample production take at least 15 minutes, and partly simple logic.

Trips away, naughty weekends in Paris or the Cotswolds or at the spa will all be fun, and improve your chances (as well as a potential name for any progeny). If you plan it out you'll be able to look forward two or three months ahead, and even during the darker times there will be bright spots ahead.

Finally for this stage: **Set a target**, and stick to it! This is an absolute.

Example: Pregnant by 12 months' time. Set a date, write it down, put it in your calendars. It's there but not a threat - it's an agreement, this is the plan. And if you don't make it you'll go to stage two, it's not the end, it's just the first step.

This doesn't need to start right now, you might want to get your eggs (sorry for the pun) in a row. Your partner might need a few months to quit or change her job, you might both need to save up while you have two incomes, and it might be Christmas coming up. I'd suggest not starting on January 1st (too much stress in December already), but February 1st isn't bad, it isn't much longer to wait. (Note: My wife's comment: "It fucking is". Even now we're not aligned…). But, to emphasise, once the date is set, and you're in it, stick to it. It's 12 months (or 15, or 18, whatever you agree), but don't change it.

Use the time before you start to plan some trips, maybe just weekend getaways, or summer chill-outs. Getting them in the diary will add to the anticipation, and start giving the entire plan structure, and solidity.

Many IVF clinics have waiting lists, and once women get on them, they often get pregnant, as mentioned before some clinics legendarily have better pregnancy rates for their waiting lists than their actual IVF cycles. This, I think, is in part because the women involved can see something is happening, they feel there is a plan. If you try and tinker with the plan, this benefit will be lost. This is not to say that life won't intervene, stuff does happen, but it needs to be really big before you risk this. If something does happen, then agree the pause and go back to the plan. And, please, please don't allow yourselves to lose heart after 6 months and rush to stage 2.

The only exception to this is if the tests show something serious which requires intervention such as an operation which may cause you to put the plan on hold, or even restart after the operation, or it may move you to Stage 2, or even 3.

Stage 2 - Medical Intervention

This is a tough stage, but one which needs to be approached together, with eyes wide open. You need to discuss and plan, and make sure you're both happy. If the answer is Clomid followed by IVF, then that's what you do. Save for it, prepare for it, and don't complain.

Just like in Stage 1, you need a plan. But this time it's how to manage the process. It is important that you, as a couple, take charge of this, it will help you avoid drifting, and avoid exacerbating the helplessness which will sometimes be overwhelming. We took three IVF cycles to really get on top of this, it made those much more painful than they needed to be.

If it's IVF, you need to know that it's a conveyor belt process, it's impersonal, it's stressful, and it may well take multiple attempts. I would suggest that if you can afford it, or get it paid for, aim for something like four cycles, three months apart.

The tricky thing here is to try not to stress over each individual cycle, even though your partner will be. Stay calm, support her, do not add to her stress load at all if you can help it. You need to be thinking that they are rolls of the dice, and if it doesn't work, that's fine, there's another one.

Even if it's the last one, then you have a plan (see next stage). Don't be worried if the gap between IVFs is four or five months, but don't squish them too closely together, the cycles are very stressful, and there is evidence that a woman's fertility is enhanced for 2-3 months after each cycle and therefore that's when you should be having sex and trying to conceive naturally.

Plan each cycle, where you will be and what you'll do. The week(s) initially after implantation are extremely stressful. Take some time off, maybe do local things you wouldn't normally do, binge-watch a series. You won't be able to get her mind off it, but you might be able to make it lighter. Cook (or order in) some nice meals, pamper her. For two reasons, 1) reducing her stress should help the process succeed, 2) it shows that you're committed and in for the long haul, which you need to show if it doesn't go well. There will be dark days, you might be finding it tough too, but man up, take it on the chin and look after her.

Know that IVFs fail. More often than not. They're just a way of increasing the odds, and reducing some of the risks (e.g. ICSI), but you need to be ready for the failure, and minimise the impact. Making it a one big roll of the dice is really not going to help. If this means you need to save money, then save money. It's better to have some money saved which you don't need to spend on another round of IVF, and can spend on a baby, then increase the likelihood of wasting an IVF round with stress (even if you are getting it free).

For each cycle, if it doesn't work, then have a plan, go somewhere nice (a day trip to the coast or the lakes, or if you can, a weekend away), it's a commiseration, but it's also a chance to be together, and look forward to the next part of the plan. You might also want to have a few things planned for the time gap till the next cycle (not all need to be big ones, a nice evening out would also be good), her fertility should be increased, and you want to be able to take advantage of that.

That also brings me to another point, sex. You should still be having it, and in the, hopefully, positive way you developed in phase 1. Not during the actual cycles of course, but before and during the gaps between cycles, if there are any. At the same frequency. Just because you're spending a lot of money on a medically enhanced shot, you shouldn't give up on the natural route.

There are also complications which might mean you need to make some tough decisions. You need to be ready for them. Some might have come up in stage 1, and you might need to consider sperm or egg donors, or perhaps surrogacy. You might have to pay for ICSI. It is so much better to talk this all through and know where you are.

Finally (and just like stage 1): **Set a target**, and stick to it!

Pregnant by 18 months' time. Four cycles with three months between each. That is the target, and if you don't make it, you'll go to stage three. This will be hard.

Stage 3 - Other options

Adoption? Fostering? Giving it all up to go sailing round the world. Finding a cave in deepest darkest Devon to hide in for six months?

The point is you gave it a really good shot, but now you need to move on. It's probably been depressing, exhausting and tearful, but you need to turn the page. It is absolutely not easy, but it is necessary.

There are tales (and you'll hear so many of them) of people adopting and then falling pregnant, or giving up and then next month it happens, but don't rely on them, whatever you do at this stage needs to be real.

I'd like to write more on this, to be of some help, but the truth is I was never ready for it. We talked about surrogacy, and even looked at the costs to do it in Thailand. What I refused to discuss, somewhat, now, to my shame, was adoption. I think I felt it would be giving up, and I was always uncomfortable with the idea in itself in a general, if somewhat nebulous, way.

You will need to support each other, and hopefully you'll have support from family and close friends. Even so, all I can say is that if you are in this place then you need to make sure you are getting help and support from mental health professionals. I know I'd have argued against this at the time, but I was entirely wrong. You have been through one of the most stressful situations in modern life. A multi-year, painful, both physically and mentally, process. It's not going to be easy, and you aren't being tough, or sensible, by not getting help from people who know how to support you.

191

5

Things I Wish I'd Known

Hindsight is always painful, but here are the things I really wish I'd known before we started...

It's Not Easy To Get Pregnant - I took away from my sex education classes that if there was a single sperm in a room with a woman not on the pill then she would get pregnant. Sperm needed to be killed by spermicide in a condom, and she should have smothered herself with spermicidal cream (preferably a lubricant version), and be on the pill. Then, and only then, might you avoid getting her pregnant, and even then, it was probably better not to do anything until marriage.

This turns out to be mostly wrong. I mean, it's probably not entirely inaccurate for 16-year olds, but once you're in your late twenties or thirties, things have become a little more complex. Even if everything is functioning, and you hit the right moment of the cycle, and you're in top condition, it's more likely than not that nothing will happen. In fact, at one point I started thinking that even having a condom in the room might be affecting our chances of conception.

There Is An Industry - there are books (like this one), specialists, tests, supplements, diets, acupuncture courses, yoga, herbs and pills, and that's before you get to Clomid, ICSI and IVF. There's a lot of noise, and a lot of it is snake oil. They're preying on the hopes and fears of desperate people. Navigating your way through this is painful (expensive), and ultimately depressing (if the latest fad doesn't work). We tried pills (at one point we were taking about a hundred different supplements a day), acupuncture, faith healing, home blood tests, blah-therapy, burning incense, having a pan-pipe music CD in the house, counselling, IVF, weekend breaks, many diets, Chinese medicine, in fact I don't even recall the whole list. After a while it became another thing to keep my wife happy. This did not endear me, as I wasn't great at hiding my scepticism (so if I wear this snake-skin around my neck for a week then my sperm will be enhanced??).

She Thinks About It All The Time - so there's an old story about men thinking about sex every ten seconds (or whatever the current variant is). The fact is, if your partner is in child purgatory, she will be thinking about wanting to have a child every ten seconds. It will be the first thing she thinks of in the morning, and the last thing at night. She will be thinking of that while shouting at you about drinking too much wine, or while commiserating with you about a bad day at the office, whatever she's doing in her life, work, sport, going out, is basically background to a constant ache. And every time you do something to poke that ache, you are not helping.

Sex Is Not Always The Answer - really. Sometimes other methods are required. Accept it. Don't fight it. This is not necessarily a comment on you.

Boasting About How Great Your Sperm Is Doesn't Help - apparently this is seen as rubbing in the fact that it is all her. Which is not going to help one little bit. It's also quite probably not entirely accurate, so it's worth getting a few tests done over the course of several months to confirm. Even if these do show that you have champion sperm... keep the knowledge and boasting to yourself!

We Don't Know A Lot - the amount we know about infertility is shockingly small. Two-thirds to three-quarters of infertility is unexplained; doctors simply don't know. This means that when you speak to someone who confidently asserts that you'll be expecting a little one soon, he or she is probably just a sale person for the Industry.

Further, **What Is Known By Some Isn't Necessarily Shared Knowledge** - we still know quite a bit, but it's not shared widely. For example, varicoceles (varicose veins on testicles) are considered likely to be bad for sperm health, and can be treated fairly simply. It was not mentioned to us by any of the experts we saw over a six year period (including two of the UK's top clinics and experts in the US). It was only through a friend of my wife's we heard about it.

You Are In Charge Of This Process – yes, the pair of you, are in charge. We're used to trusting doctors and letting them lead, but in this case (other than where treatment is required for medical reasons) you are not a patient, you're a customer, and therefore you need to be in charge. Ask questions, research things, say no, demand treatment, whatever it is, do not let someone else force you along a process you don't like, don't want to go down, or don't think will work.

She Is In Purgatory - the concept of purgatory as a relentless waiting place before heaven has always seem somewhat despicable to me. And worse, like many words it has become debased by continuous use. However, it is an apt description of the state of many women who are trying, and currently failing, to become pregnant.

If somebody could sit them down and say, "Look, it'll take 7 years, but then you'll have a child," then many of them, except perhaps the most competitive, would relax, and accept it. But they don't know. They don't know if it will take 6 months, a year, five years or never, and it's continuous and real. Their biological clocks are ticking loudly and continuously, and they don't know if that clock will stop ticking before they have a baby.

It's worse than that though. We live in an instant gratification society (pretty much everyone reading this in English anyway), we want something, we buy it. Perhaps we might have to save up, or borrow, but mostly things happen. New iphone? Done. That new clothing item. Done. Easy credit. Anything. But biology, it doesn't play by those rules. It runs to its own beat, and as yet we can do very little to influence that. But culturally we are not attuned to that, so finally coming up against something which can't be bought or cajoled into happening makes it even worse for many women.

The lack of control is the most painful aspect of the situation. There are no levers which will instantly make her pregnant, and after months or years of trying this can become all consuming.

And then ...

Two years later, in a fit of crazy enthusiasm, we decided to give it another go. There had been that conversation, nine years before, in that crazy jokey way you do, that we both always fancied having four. So, another go it was (well two to be exact). I was in a different world. I had been pregnant, I had seen, with my own eyes, my own positive pregnancy test. After the first IVF failed, we tried, "one last time" and there it was again – that life giving faint blue line. It was the same MO, no belly rubbing, big proper pregnancy clothes, lying on the left every night and thanking my lucky stars that I was still pregnant. Nine months later, perfectly on time, the most gorgeous, beautiful baby boy popped out. No ICU this time, he just lay in my arms all night as I stared at him in wonder and awe.

We did actually also try to use the frozen ones, so I underwent a frozen shorter cycle which seemed like a breeze compared to IVF, but on the morning they were supposed to be put back in the clinic called just as I was getting in the car to say they had never seen anything like it before but none of them were viable.

So that was it. Despite the crazy dream of four; no more IVF, no more trying. Not that I really thought about it but there was also no need for the pill, after all we hadn't been using any form of contraception for 11 years and there hadn't been even a single whiff of pregnancy in all that time.

Life moved on, we had three awesome, growing children to look after, we moved country, tried to live a more "relaxed" life (ha ha).

And then, two years later, I started trying to remember when I had last had a period. I don't really know what made me think of it. Something just felt different.

I went on a business trip and told myself if I still hadn't had a period by the time I got back, however ridiculous the notion, I would do a pregnancy test. I got back. I did a pregnancy test.

There it was again. That awesome, life confirming faint blue line.

You hear those stories all the time, unexplained fertility, stopped trying/went on holiday/got horribly drunk and wham – there's a baby. I never in my wildest dreams thought that would be me, ever. It had been ELEVEN YEARS. Eleven years of no contraception. Eleven years of desperately, desperately trying to get pregnant and not a single pregnancy in sight. And yet, another nine months later (well actually seven as it had taken me so long to work it out), there he was, a gorgeous little miracle smiling up at me. That dream all those years before had become reality. People passing us in the street now probably think I'm one of those super fertile women who just wants to have lots of babies – the latter is true but the former couldn't be further from the truth.

When I was desperately trying to get pregnant, I read as many books by people struggling with infertility as I could get my hands on. I was always tempted to start by skipping to the back, mostly hoping there was a happy ending which would give me some hope and courage to carry on but also if it was a baby-filled ending, that maybe within the pages might lie the answer, the secret, the way through the maze, to finally catch the swinging toy at the carousel.

I still don't fully understand what the secret is and I don't think there is one solution which fits all but, hopefully, within these pages you have been able to take some comfort from the fact that someone else has been on the same journey and made it through. If I could give you one piece of advice it would be this: never, ever give up. You may not be able to have a biological child, you may have to make fundamental changes to your life, you may need help and treatment (whether for mental illness, a physical problem or both), you may encounter doctors and medical professionals who are utterly useless and won't or can't help, in which case you need to find ones who can and will, you may need to reassess who you are and your relationships, you may have to fight like you've never fought for something before, you may need to beg, borrow and steal (okay maybe not the last part) but if motherhood is fundamentally what matters, if being a mother is a visceral force which is driving your every waking moment, I believe there is a way. Trust your instincts. Find your way.

AFTERWORD

As a lawyer all the proofreading errors are mine and not Jason's, so mea culpa. As a lawyer, I have also lost all ability to speak or write normally (see above) so thank you to anyone who has got this far and stuck with my rambling thoughts. Go and get a cup of tea, or some chocolate or whatever your go-to thing is, and pat yourself on the back. I hope, even in a very small way, that this book has helped you and you too find a way through to success and happiness.

To my parents, thank you for being my inspiration and my never-ending support. If I can be even a smidgin of the parent you have been to me, I will consider it a job well done.

Jason, on that fateful day in 2002, I told you there wasn't a hope in hell of me obeying you but I promised to always love, respect and support you and occasionally to try and listen to you. I am so sorry for the hell I put you through but we made it, we got through it and came out the other side, still together, still taking the piss. You are, and always will be, the voice in my head, my rock and the love of my life.

To the GBs and the IFs. I love you more than you can possibly imagine. I still pinch myself and say thank you every day that you are here. Wow, what a journey but it was so, so worth it.